RISE™

Body Trust, Movement, & Mindful Strength

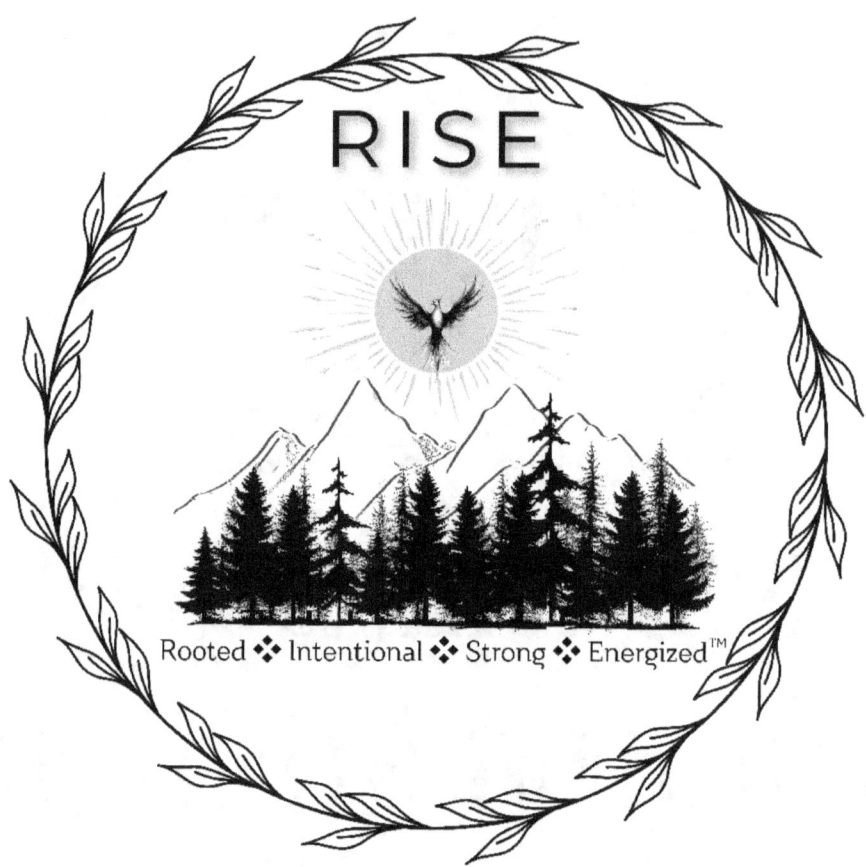

RISE

Rooted ❖ Intentional ❖ Strong ❖ Energized™

A transformational book series

exploring balance, belief, and embodied wholeness.

RISE™

Body Trust, Movement, & Mindful Strength

Living a Rooted, Intentional, Strong, and Energized Life —

through Embodied Strength and Trust

Volume 2

Angel Tate Keaton

Healthy in Heart Media™, LLC
Roanoke, VA

Published in the United States of America by
Healthy in Heart Media™, LLC
P.O. Box 694
Vinton, VA 24179
Copyright © 2026 by Angel Tate Keaton
First Printing February 2026
Cover art and design by the author

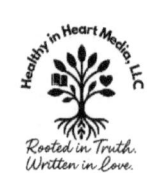

Library of Congress Control Number: 2026903976

ISBN— 978-1-969064-21-0

Trademark Notice

RISE Rooted, Intentional, Strong, Energized™, and related marks and program names are trademarks of Healthy in Heart Media, LLC. Unauthorized use is prohibited.

Disclaimer

The author of this book does not dispense medical advice or prescribe the use of any technique as a form of treatment for medical, emotional, psychological, or physical conditions without the guidance of a licensed physician or qualified healthcare provider, either directly or indirectly. The intent of the author is solely to offer information of a general nature to support you in your personal journey toward emotional, physical, mental, and spiritual well-being.

If you choose to apply any of the information presented in this book, you do so of your own volition. The author and the publisher assume no responsibility for your actions or any consequences that may arise from the use or misuse of the information contained herein.

No Guarantee of Outcomes
The practices and concepts presented in this book are intended to support whole-being wellness. Individual experiences and results may vary. The author and publisher make no guarantees regarding any specific physical, emotional, or spiritual outcomes resulting from the application of this material.

Educational Purpose Notice
This book is provided for general informational and educational purposes only and is not intended as a substitute for professional medical, psychological, counseling, or therapeutic care.

Emergency Help Notice
This material is not intended for crises. If you are experiencing a medical, mental-health, or safety emergency, contact local emergency services or a licensed professional immediately.

No Professional Relationship Notice
Reading this book does not establish a counseling, coaching, therapeutic, or professional relationship between the reader and the author or publisher. This material is for personal growth and educational use only and is not a substitute for individualized professional advice, diagnosis, or treatment.

Spiritual Disclaimer
Spiritual references and practices presented in this book reflect the author's personal faith and are offered for reflection, not as doctrinal instruction or religious authority.

Scripture Notice
Unless otherwise noted, all Scripture quotations are taken from the American Standard Version (ASV), as provided by BibleGateway.com. The American Standard Version was originally published in 1901 and is now in the public domain. This version was chosen for its consistent use of the divine name in the Old Testament and its closer alignment with the original Hebrew, making it a suitable foundation for a return-to-Eden perspective.

Dedication

For those who were taught to control their bodies
instead of listening to them.

May this book support your remembering—
that strength can be gentle,
trust can be rebuilt,
and your body is worthy of care exactly as it is.

Rise each day like the sun—

Rooted in truth,

Intentional in habits,

Strong in spirit, and

Energized for the hope of tomorrow.

~Angel Tate Keaton

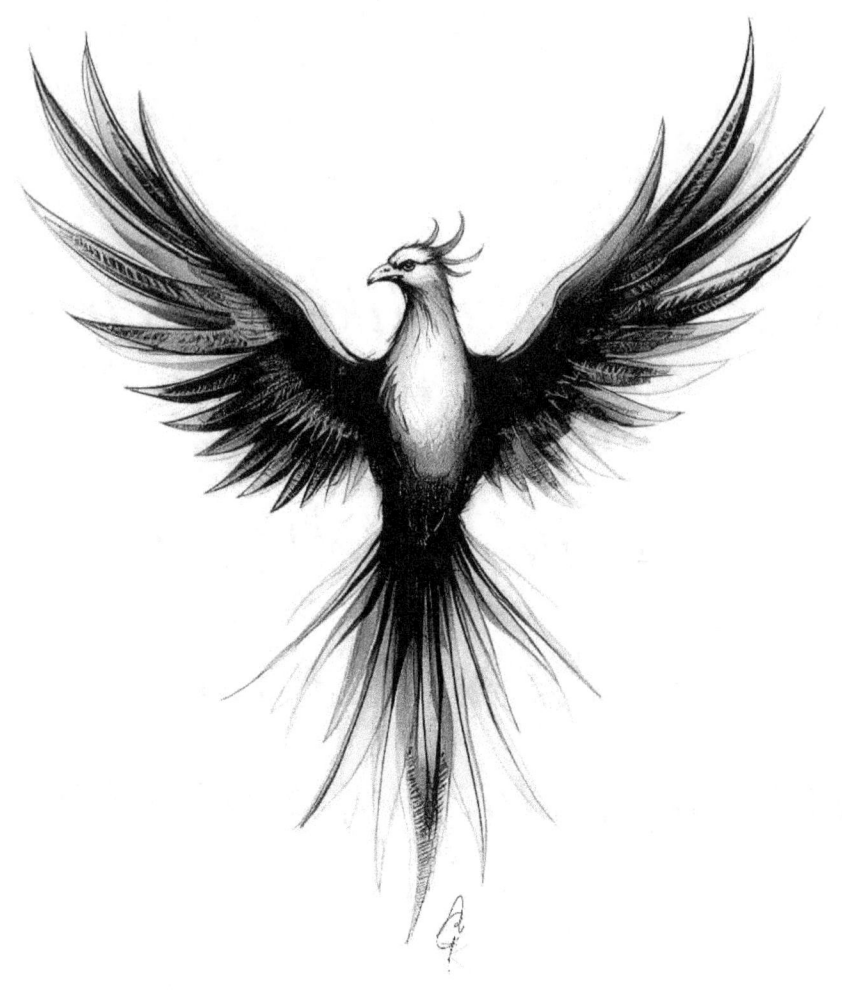

When the phoenix burns,
It does not perish.
It rises from the ashes—refined.

Table of Contents

Preface — Why I Wrote This Book

I did not write this book because movement was missing from my life.

I wrote it because trust was.

For a long time, movement existed in my world—but it no longer felt neutral, joyful, or safe. It became something to manage, optimize, or endure. Like many people, I learned to move in ways that prioritized outcomes over my relationship with my body, disciplining it versus listening to it, and appearance over presence. Over time, the cost of that approach became clear—not just in my body, but in how I related to myself.

This book was born out of that reckoning.

I wrote it because I saw how easily well-intended health efforts can quietly become another form of self-override. How movement meant to support life can become something we perform against our own bodies. How the language of "strength" can drift into pressure, and how shame can hide beneath even the most disciplined of routines.

I also wrote this book because I learned—slowly, and sometimes painfully—that the body is not an obstacle to overcome. It is a communicator. A carrier of memory. A witness to our lives. And when it stops responding the way we expect, it is often not because it has failed us, but because it has been asking to be heard.

There were seasons when injury, burnout, and medical realities forced me to stop approaching movement the way I always had. At first, that felt like a loss. Over time, it became an invitation to rethink strength, redefine progress, and rebuild trust not through force but through consistency, compassion, and respect.

What surprised me most was how much my identity shifted alongside the physical changes. As I stopped pushing and started listening, I noticed that my relationship with my body softened—and so did my relationship with myself. Movement became less about fixing and more about participating. Care replaced control. Trust replaced fear.

This book is not a program. It is not a prescription. And it is not written to tell you what your body *should* be capable of.

It is written to help you listen.

Across these pages, I explore movement not as a performance, but as a relationship. Strength not as domination, but as support. Progress not as a number, but as lived experience. The goal is not to arrive at a perfected body, but to inhabit the one you have with greater safety, presence, and respect.

I wrote this book for anyone who has ever felt disconnected from their body.

For anyone whose movement history includes injury, shame, burnout, or confusion.

For anyone who wants to care for their body without turning it into a project.

Most of all, I wrote it because I believe healing does not begin with pushing harder.

It begins with trust.

And trust—when rebuilt patiently—is a complete game changer.

Acknowledgments

To the women of the RISE Momentum Circle—you are the living echo of this work and the steady inspiration behind every page.

Thank you for your honesty, your courage, and your willingness to walk toward wholeness together.

Your presence has shaped this message more than you know.

To my husband, Todd—thank you for believing in me long before I learned how to do so myself.

Your patience, grounded love, and quiet strength have been a constant anchor and a gentle lift.

To the teachers, mentors, and healers who poured truth into my life—thank you for pointing me toward freedom when fear tried to set the limits.

Your guidance helped me recognize what was always available.

To every person who offered kindness, clarity, or hope along the way—your words are woven into these pages, whether you know it or not.

And above all, to my Creator—thank You for breath, for belonging, and for the balance You designed from the beginning.

May this work reflect Your wisdom and honor the wholeness You intended.

With profound gratitude,
Angel Tate Keaton

How to Use This Book

This book is designed to support your whole-being wellness—body, mind, emotions, and spirit—one week at a time, with particular attention to movement, body trust, and embodied strength. There is no rush, no falling behind, and no "right" way to move through it. There is only your pace and your presence.

This is a guided journey, not a demand. Let it meet you where you are—in the body you have today.

Your Personal Journey

Most readers will walk this path individually, using the weekly rhythm as a steady companion for reflection, reconnection, and sustainable movement. Even when you are engaging this work on your own, you are not alone. Many others are exploring these same themes—learning to listen to their bodies with greater respect, patience, and trust.

This book is meant to be a safe place to notice, feel, and grow—without performance, comparison, or pressure.

Optional Guided Connection

If you are interested in participating in an author-led RISE Momentum Circle, you may request more information directly. These guided spaces, when available, are facilitated by the creator of this work and are designed to remain grounded, trauma-informed, and rooted in encouragement rather than instruction or therapy.

Participation is always optional, and availability may vary. This book is complete and supportive as a standalone journey.

If you'd like to explore current or future RISE Momentum Circle offerings, you can visit: https://healthyinheart.com/rise-wellness-community

Your Weekly Rhythm in This Book

Each week centers on one embodied theme and includes:

1. A short chapter offering perspective, context, and lived wisdom
2. Reflection prompts that help translate insight into body awareness
3. One gentle focus practice to support integration without overwhelm

4. A RISE Check-In to notice what is strengthening, softening, or asking for care

Simple. Steady. Sustainable.

Pairing With the RISE Journal

This book is part of the *RISE Circle of Wholeness Collection.*

The companion journal supports daily integration through:

> guided reflection spaces

> breath and body-awareness prompts

> weekly acknowledgments of growth

> visual reminders of rhythm, ritual, and rest

If you are using both together, this book offers the why—the journal supports the how.

A Trauma-Informed Journey

Healing should never feel forced.

Throughout this book, you will find invitations—not requirements. You are always free to:

> skip a prompt

> take more time

> pause when emotions or sensations feel intense

> return when your body feels ready

Your nervous system is your guide.
Honor what feels safe, spacious, and supportive.

This journey is about restoration, not endurance.

A Final Word Before We Begin

Wholeness isn't something that happens all at once.
It grows slowly—like becoming *Real*.*

Shaped by honesty, softened by love,
and strengthened every time you choose to stay present
instead of disappearing.

You don't become whole through perfection—
you become whole by being **fully here**:
scuffs, scars, beauty, and all.

So, take a deep breath.
You're not stepping into performance—
you're stepping into presence.
Each small choice, each loving moment,
brings you one step closer to a more
authentic, embodied, beautifully Real **you**.

Welcome to your next rise.
Let's begin

* *This reflection is lovingly inspired by the conversation on becoming "Real" from*
The Velveteen Rabbit *by Margery Williams (1922).*

Overview of the RISE Framework

A Pathway Back to Whole-Being Wellness

RISE is more than a wellness model—it is a return to the way we were created to live:

Rooted • Intentional • Strong • Energized

Every person rises through four dimensions—body, mind, spirit, and community—each intertwined like threads in a tapestry of wholeness. Before we reshape habits or rebuild rhythms, we begin with identity.

Identity steadies the ground beneath us so change can take root. That is why Identity & Worth Volume 1 introduces the RISE way of living by anchoring you in who you truly are, long before we expand into deeper lifestyle practices in future volumes.

The RISE Framework gives language, symbols, and gentle practices that begin transforming daily life one small, meaningful shift at a time.

R — Rooted

Rooted people are steady, grounded, nourished, and connected.

Circumstances, labels, or storms do not define them, because their identity is anchored in something deeper and more eternal.

To be rooted is to live from truth—not reaction.

Rootedness looks like:

Strong internal foundations

Eating what nourishes the body

Slowing down enough to listen

Returning to who you are beneath old labels

Choosing connection over chaos

Rooted people grow with confidence because they are not afraid of being uprooted.

I — Intentional

Intentional living means moving through life with clarity, purpose, and conscious choice.

It is the opposite of drifting, numbing, or living from inherited beliefs.

Intentionality expresses itself through:

> Mindfulness in daily decisions
>
> Choosing rather than reacting
>
> Creating rhythms instead of chasing urgency
>
> Speaking truth with compassion
>
> Aligning actions with deeply held values

Intentional people move with meaning—even in the smallest moments.

S — Strong

Strength is not force.

It is integrity, emotional steadiness, and inner resilience.

It is the capacity to stay rooted in truth even when life shakes the ground.

RISE strength includes:

> Emotional stability
>
> Boundaries that honor self and others
>
> Courage to speak and choose wisely

Resilience in adversity

A balanced confidence

Willingness to heal and grow

Strength allows you to face life with a steady heart and a grounded identity.

E — Energized

Energized living is not a frantic hustle or endless output.

It is sustainable, life-giving vitality—the natural fruit of alignment, nourishment, and inner freedom.

Energized people experience:

Joy that flows without force

Rhythms of work and rest that restore

Clarity instead of overwhelm

Purpose without burnout

A sense of internal lightness

This is what it means to be fully alive.

The Circle of Wholeness

A Whole-System View of Human Flourishing

The Circle of Wholeness is the visual model that holds the entire RISE ecosystem.

It teaches that wellness is not linear—it is circular, interconnected, and dynamic.

In the Circle:

> Every area of life impacts every other
>
> Small choices ripple outward
>
> Minor shifts create meaningful healing

You cannot "fix" one area without touching the whole.

The Circle of Wholeness includes Nine Pillars, each represented by a nature-based symbol.

These symbols are simple, universal, and spiritually resonant—giving every participant a way to connect with truth no matter their background.

The Nine Pillars of Wholeness

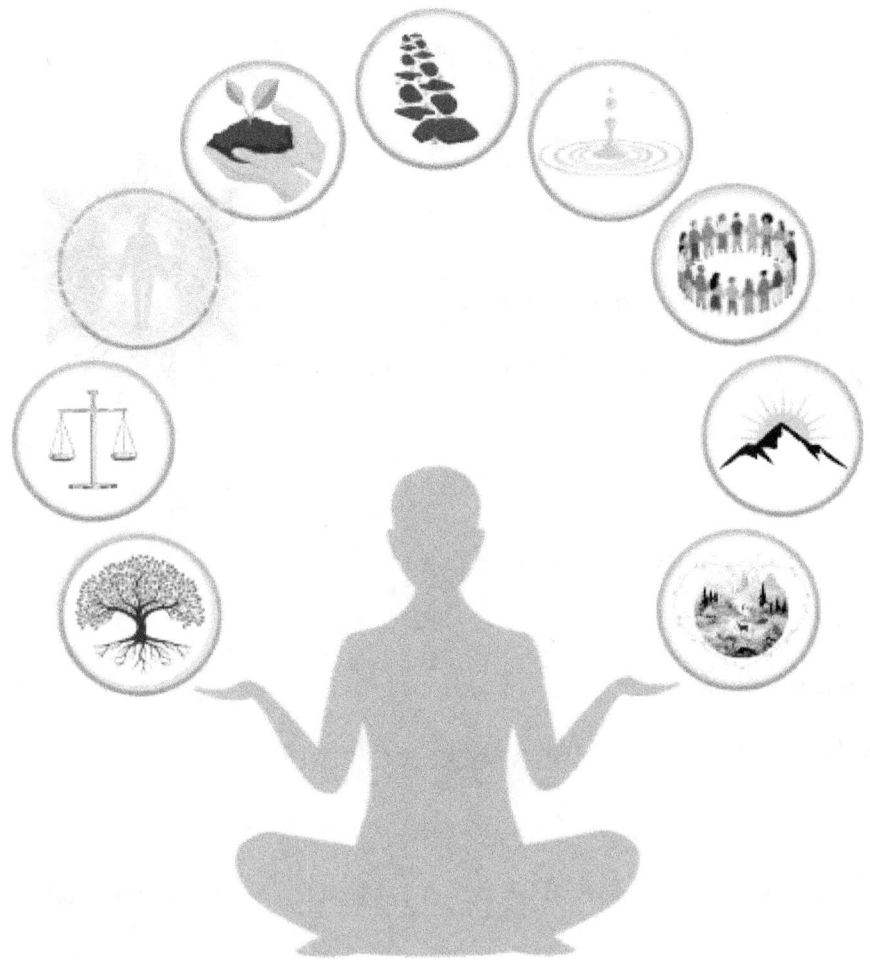

Each pillar includes its symbol, meaning, practice, and reflection question.

1. The Tree of Life — Rooted Health

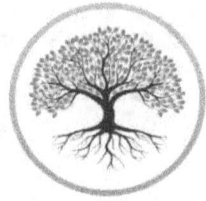

Meaning: Connection, nourishment, vitality.

Wholeness begins underground: strong roots create strong lives.

Practice:

    Eat from creation (living foods)

    Move with gratitude

    Rest before exhaustion

Reflection: What keeps my roots strong today?

2. The Scales of Balance — Living in Alignment

Meaning: Harmony across body, mind, spirit, and relationships.

Balance is alignment, not perfection.

Practice:

Pause midday to breathe and recenter

Simplify one crowded area

Reflection: Where can I recalibrate gently instead of striving?

3. The Radiant Human — Flowing Energy Within

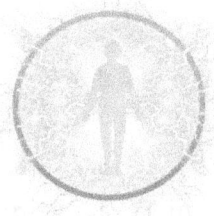

Meaning: Inner light and vitality flow when beliefs, thoughts, and spirit agree.

Practice:

Begin with three deep breaths

Practice prayer, meditation, or mindful movement

Reflection: How can I let my inner light guide my pace?

4. Hands of Stewardship — Nurturing What's Given

Meaning: Responsibility, gratitude, tending what has been entrusted.

Practice:

Do one act of care (body, home, relationship)

Offer encouragement or gratitude

Reflection: What am I stewarding with love today?

5. The Garden Path — Healing as a Journey

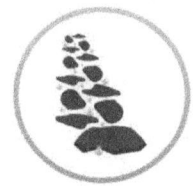

Meaning: Healing is not linear; it unfolds over time.

Practice:

Notice progress without judgment

Rest purposefully once a week

Reflection: What is today teaching me about patience?

6. The Water Ripple — The Power of Small Choices

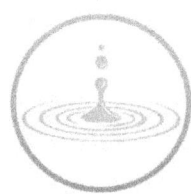

Meaning: Every choice sends ripples into the whole.

Practice:

Make one nourishing choice

Notice its ripple into mood and relationships

Reflection: How can one small shift bring wider peace?

7. The Circle of People — Healing Together

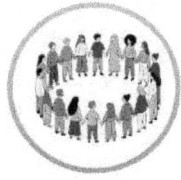

Meaning: We heal in community, not isolation.

Practice:

    Reach out to encourage

    Ask for help when needed

Reflection: Who forms my circle of support?

8. Sunrise Over Mountains — Renewal & Hope

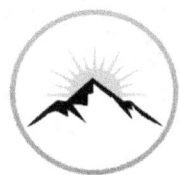

Meaning: Dawn after darkness; every day a new beginning.

Practice:

    Start with gratitude

    Reframe setbacks as sunrise lessons

Reflection: Where do I see new light emerging?

9. The Heart in Creation — Love at the Center

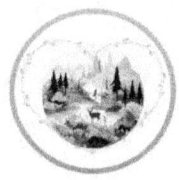

Meaning: Love sustains the ecosystem of wholeness—compassion, unity, divine rhythm.

Practice:

Speak kindness to yourself and others

Do one act of care for creation

Reflection: How can I let love move through me today?

How the RISE Framework, Circle of Wholeness & Nine Pillars Work Together

Together, these three layers form an integrated ecosystem of transformation:

RISE™ — The Four Qualities of a Whole Person

Rooted • Intentional • Strong • Energized

These are the inner postures that shape how you move through the world.

The Circle of Wholeness — The Whole-Life Model

An interconnected system where physical, emotional, relational, and spiritual well-being support one another.

The Nine Pillars — The Daily Practices

Simple, repeatable habits that create sustainable change over time.

Together, they help you:

Remember your worth

Heal body, mind, and spirit

Reconnect with community

Establish nourishing rhythms

Develop emotional stability

Return to the Creator's design

Transform from within

This is the foundation of your Identity & Worth journey—a return to who you were made to be.

Chapter 1 — Joyful Movement & Body Trust

Movement did not always feel complicated.

For a long time, it was simply something I did because I loved it. I ran—not to burn something off or prove discipline, but because it felt freeing. Running gave me space. It gave me rhythm. It gave me joy. There was something deeply grounding about the steady cadence of breath and feet, the way movement carried my thoughts without demanding explanation.

That changed the moment movement became something I had to do instead of something I wanted to do.

After tearing the medial meniscus in my left knee, I was told I could no longer run. The injury itself was painful, but the loss that followed was deeper. Recovery required surgery, and that season was traumatic in ways that lingered long after the knee healed. My relationship with my body changed—not because my body failed me, but because I was suddenly unsure whether I could trust it.

That uncertainty can be more destabilizing than the pain itself.

Many people know this moment. Not always through running, but through injury, illness, diagnosis, pregnancy, aging, trauma, or limitation. The moment when movement stops feeling neutral or joyful and starts feeling fragile, conditional, or restricted. When the body no longer feels predictable, trust quietly erodes.

When that happens, movement often shifts without our consent.

It becomes cautious. Calculated. Managed.

And eventually, it can become something we perform against the body rather than with it.

When Movement Becomes About Control

I did not use movement as punishment, but I did begin to use it as a tool for weight loss in unhealthy ways. The focus narrowed. The metrics grew louder. Movement stopped being relational and became transactional.

Instead of asking how movement felt, I began asking what it produced. Calories. Minutes. Progress. Outcomes.

Over time, my body pushed back—not through rebellion, but through burnout. There came a season where anything felt like punishment, even movement I once enjoyed. Exhaustion replaced motivation. What was once life-giving became draining, not because movement itself was wrong, but because the framework around it had become rigid and demanding.

This is how disconnection often forms—not through obvious self-harm, but through well-intended striving that ignores the body's limits.

Burnout is not laziness.

It is not a lack of discipline.

It is the body asking to be listened to.

When movement becomes something we use to control outcomes—weight, worth, or approval—it loses its capacity to restore. The nervous system stays on alert. The body braces. Joy disappears, not because the body is incapable of joy, but because it no longer feels safe.

How the Body Learns to Distrust Movement

The body remembers how it is treated.

When movement consistently follows guilt, fear, or pressure, the body learns to associate movement with threat rather than care. Even well-intended routines can become sources of tension if they override hunger, exhaustion, pain, or emotional needs.

This is especially true for those who have experienced trauma, medical loss, or chronic stress. The body's signals may have been ignored for survival. Pushing through may once have been necessary. But survival strategies, when carried too long, become sources of harm.

Disconnection is not failure.

It is an adaptation.

Understanding this reframes the work ahead. Rebuilding body trust is not about correcting a broken system. It is about gently restoring communication with your body, which adapted to keep you safe.

Movement as Relationship, Not Rule

Rebuilding body trust begins when movement is no longer treated as something to control the body, but as something done with the body.

The body does not experience movement as punishment unless it is taught to. Before numbers, trackers, and expectations, movement was simply part of being alive—walking, stretching, carrying, resting, dancing. It was responsive, not prescriptive.

When movement is relational, the body responds differently. There is less resistance. Less bracing. More cooperation. Joyful movement feels life-giving rather than draining. It reconnects us with a sense of presence rather than pressure.

For me, joy now shows up in walking, dancing, gentle Pilates, and light strength work—forms of movement that feel safe to my nervous system and respectful of my body's realities.

Joy is not about intensity.

It is about resonance.

Movement that brings joy often reconnects us with earlier experiences—before performance entered the picture. Before movement was evaluated, instead of being felt. When time passed quickly because the body was engaged, not judged.

Listening to the Body's Real Constraints

Part of rebuilding trust has meant honoring medical realities instead of pushing past them.

I live with pigment dispersion syndrome, a condition in which pigment granules from the iris can block eye drainage, leading to increased intraocular pressure and raising the risk of glaucoma. Certain activities—such as intense weight lifting, high-impact exercise, or positions where the head is lowered for extended periods (common in yoga and Pilates)—can exacerbate pressure changes in the eyes.

This means my body has clear boundaries.

Honoring those boundaries is not weakness.

It is wisdom.

So many people are taught that limits mean failure—that modification equals quitting. But real care requires discernment. The body is not asking to be dominated. It is asking to be protected.

Listening to the body means noticing patterns—fatigue, tension, restlessness, emotional shifts—and responding with care instead of correction. Some days that means movement. Other days it means rest. Trust grows not by getting it right every time, but by responding consistently with respect.

The Role of the Nervous System in Joyful Movement

Joyful movement is not just about muscles and joints. It is deeply tied to nervous system safety.

When the nervous system feels threatened—by pressure, comparison, pain, or fear—movement becomes guarded. The body braces. Breath shortens. Joy becomes inaccessible.

When the nervous system feels safe, movement softens. Breath deepens. Curiosity returns.

This is why slowing down matters. Why gentle movement can be more healing than intense effort. Why walking, stretching, or dancing can restore connection faster than pushing through another routine.

Safety is the soil where joy grows.

Intuitive Movement Is Compassionate Wisdom

Intuitive movement does not mean abandoning structure or accountability. It means applying wisdom with compassion.

There was a time when strict plans felt safer than listening inwardly. Letting go of rigidity brought fear—fear of losing progress, fear of doing "too little," fear of slipping back. Those fears are understandable. They deserve gentleness, not judgment.

Intuition grows through curiosity. By asking, "What does my body need today?" rather than "What should I force myself to do?"

Some days, that answer is strength.

Some days, it is stretching.

Some days, it is walking slowly.

And some days it is rest without explanation.

Intuitive movement challenges all-or-nothing thinking. It allows flexibility without guilt. It honors the reality that bodies change from day to day—and that wisdom adapts.

Strength Reimagined

Strength used to mean endurance.

Pushing.

Ignoring discomfort.

Now, strength means something different.

It means the ability to respond rather than react. To rest without guilt. To move with intention. To stop when stopping is wise. To remain connected to the body instead of overriding it.

Strength is no longer measured by how much I can tolerate.

It is measured by how well I can listen.

True strength supports life. It does not dominate the body.

One of the most healing moments in this journey came when it was gently pointed out to me that my body has carried me through my entire life—through injuries, illness, and many forms of abuse I pushed myself through—and yet it still shows up for me every day.

That realization shifted my perspective in a very important way.

My body was never the enemy.

It was faithful.

Grief, Gratitude, and Reconciliation

Rebuilding body trust often includes grief.

Grief for what was lost.

For abilities that changed.

For seasons that demanded endurance instead of care.

Grief does not negate gratitude. The two can coexist. In fact, gratitude often deepens when it grows alongside grief.

Honoring what the body has endured—and what it still offers—creates space for reconciliation. Not a forced positivity, but a grounded respect for the body's persistence.

This reconciliation is not instantaneous. It unfolds through daily choices that say, I am listening now.

A New Invitation

This chapter is not about fixing movement.

It is about restoring the relationship.

It is about releasing the belief that movement must be earned, intense, or corrective. It is about learning to listen again. About honoring real limitations without shame. About redefining strength as connection rather than control.

Movement was never meant to be a battleground.

It was meant to be a conversation.

And conversations begin with *listening*.

Journal Prompts

When did movement begin to feel complicated for you, and what changed in your relationship with your body during that time?

As you write, consider:

>What movement once felt like before expectations or pressure entered the picture

>What your body may have been protecting you from

>What trust feels like now, even if it is still fragile

Write without trying to fix anything. This is about witnessing, not resolving.

What messages has your body learned about movement — and which of those messages are you ready to question?

You might reflect on:

>Whether movement has felt like care, control, obligation, or safety

>How your nervous system responds when you think about moving

>What your body seems to need in order to feel safe again

There is no right answer — only honest noticing.

If your body could speak honestly about movement, what would it want you to know right now?

Let the response come slowly.

You are not required to agree — only to listen.

Chapter 2 — Making Movement a Lifestyle

For many of us, movement framed as exercise failed not because we lacked discipline, but because it was presented as a separate event rather than a way of living.

It was scheduled, tracked, optimized, and evaluated—often in short bursts of intensity followed by long stretches of burnout. When life became complicated, movement was the first thing to disappear, reinforcing the belief that consistency requires ideal conditions.

But movement was never meant to *compete* with real life.

It was meant to be woven into it.

A movement lifestyle is not built through perfection. It is built through rhythm— through practices that adapt across seasons, energy levels, health realities, and responsibilities. When movement becomes part of *how we live* rather than *something we perform*, it stops collapsing under pressure.

This chapter is an invitation to stop asking, "How can I fit movement into my life?"

And start asking, "How can movement live where my life already is?"

Why Most Movement Plans Collapse

Most movement plans are designed for ideal circumstances.

They assume consistent energy, predictable schedules, stable health, and uninterrupted motivation. They are built around what should work rather than what does work.

So, when real life intervenes—illness, caregiving, emotional exhaustion, workload, hormonal shifts—the plan breaks. And when the plan breaks, many people assume they are the problem.

This is not a discipline issue.

Let me repeat that: This is NOT a discipline issue.

It is a design flaw.

Movement systems that only function under perfect conditions are fragile by definition. Sustainable movement must be resilient enough to survive imperfect days, interrupted weeks, and changing seasons of life.

A lifestyle adapts.

A performance collapses.

What "Realistic" Actually Means

A realistic movement routine is not one that looks good on paper. It is one that fits the life you are actually living—not the life you imagine having someday.

For a long time, I believed consistency required sameness. That every day needed to look roughly the same for movement to "count." That belief quietly set me up for failure. As soon as energy dipped, health shifted, or life demanded more, the routine broke—and with it, my sense of trust.

Consistency didn't come when I tried harder.

It came when I loosened my grip.

Now, a realistic routine leaves room for flexibility. Some days that means walking. Other days, it means stretching, gentle strength, or mindful movement. When I stopped expecting every day to look the same, movement finally became something I could return to instead of something I abandoned.

Sustainability matters so much more than intensity. **Always.**

Realistic movement is not lazy movement.

It is livable movement.

Rhythm Over Rigid Structure

A lifestyle is built through rhythm, not rules.

Rhythm allows for variation. It recognizes that bodies are cyclical, not mechanical. Energy fluctuates. Needs shift. Capacity expands and contracts.

Rigid structure demands sameness regardless of context. Rhythm responds to context.

When movement follows rhythm, it becomes easier to return to. There is no "falling off" because there is no narrow track to fall from—only a relationship that continues.

Rhythm says: This looks different today, and that's okay.

Rules say: This only counts if it looks the same.

The body responds better to rhythm.

Movement on Hard Days

Hard days tell the truth about our relationship with movement.

On those days, the old rules often surface:

> If you can't do it properly, don't do it at all.

> If you don't have energy, you're failing.

> Rest is weakness.

But hard days require gentleness, not self-punishment.

Movement on a difficult day might look like a short walk, light stretching, or even a few minutes of mindful breathing. It might look like staying connected rather than checking a box. These choices maintain continuity—and continuity builds trust.

Lowering the bar on purpose has been one of the most protective decisions I've ever made. It has kept me from quitting entirely. It has reminded my body that movement is safe, supportive, and responsive—not demanding.

Sometimes movement helps regulate emotion.

Sometimes rest is the regulation.

Learning the difference is part of the work.

Why Lowering the Bar Is Not Failure

Lowering the bar is often misunderstood as giving up when, in reality, it is an act of wisdom. When the bar is set too high, avoidance grows. Then shame follows. Eventually, movement disappears altogether. Lowering the bar keeps the relationship intact.

A five-minute walk on a hard day is not a consolation prize. It is a signal of commitment.

It says: I'm still here. I'm still listening.

That consistency—quiet, imperfect, and unremarkable—is what builds trust over time.

The Habits That Actually Stick

The movement habits that last are rarely the most impressive. They are the ones that feel natural.

Walking has been the easiest habit for me to maintain, not because it is superior, but because it fits into real life. It requires no special equipment, no perfect conditions, and no performance threshold. It meets me where I am.

Hear this: Simplicity is not a compromise. It is a strategy.

When movement is easy to access, it becomes easier to return to. Environmental cues—comfortable shoes by the door, a familiar route, music that invites motion—support consistency without relying on willpower.

Instead of constantly reinventing movement, lifestyle change grows best by building on what already works.

Complexity often impresses the mind.

Simplicity sustains the body.

Environment Shapes Behavior More Than Motivation

We often blame motivation when movement doesn't happen, but motivation is unreliable. Environment is not.

Where your shoes live.

What your mornings look like.

How your space invites or resists movement.

These details matter more than intention.

A lifestyle is supported by cues that make movement feel normal, not heroic. When movement is integrated into daily life, it requires less decision-making—and therefore less resistance.

When Resistance Shows Up

Resistance is often misinterpreted as laziness; however, in reality, it usually signals overwhelm. When resistance appears, forcing compliance often backfires.

Curiosity works better than control.

I've learned to negotiate with myself rather than battle. I tell myself I'll move for five minutes and reassess. Often, starting gently dissolves the resistance. And when it doesn't, I listen. Rest without guilt is still an act of trust.

Resistance doesn't always come from the body. Often it comes from the mind—old beliefs about what movement must look like to count. Lowering expectations can break the cycle of avoidance and shame.

The first small step is usually the hardest—and the most powerful.

Rewriting the Inner Rules

Many of us carry unspoken rules about movement:

- If it's not hard, it doesn't count.
- If it's not tracked, it's pointless.
- If you stop, you've failed.

These rules keep movement brittle. They make it easy to abandon when life shifts.

A movement lifestyle replaces rules with principles:

- Stay connected.
- Respond honestly.
- Return without shame.

Principles adapt. Rules punish.

Tracking Without Losing the Relationship

Tracking movement can be helpful, but it can also be harmful.

Data can increase awareness, but it can also turn movement into a transaction—something done for numbers instead of nourishment. There have been seasons where tracking helped me notice patterns, and seasons where it quietly fed pressure and judgment.

The problem is not data.

The problem is when data becomes the authority.

Now, I am selective. I track only what supports awareness, not what creates anxiety. Some seasons benefit from structure. Others benefit from release. Wisdom is in knowing the difference.

Movement is a relationship first. Tools should *serve* that relationship—not *replace* it.

Seasons Change. So Should Movement.

A lifestyle assumes change. Bodies age. Health shifts. Responsibilities shrink and grow. Energy fluctuates. A movement system that cannot adapt to these realities will not last.

Seasonal movement allows intensity to rise and fall. It allows focus to shift. It honors recovery as part of progress.

This is not an inconsistency. It is maturity.

Living, Not Performing

Movement becomes a lifestyle when it supports your life instead of competing with it.

It adapts.

It softens.

It stays present through change.

It does **not** demand ideal conditions to exist.

A lifestyle is built through returning—again and again—without shame.

Consistency is not doing the same thing every day.

Consistency is staying connected over time.

And when movement is allowed to live where you live—inside your real days, your real body, your real limits—it becomes something you can carry forward, season after season.

Journal Prompts

Where has movement felt like something you had to "fit in" rather than something that lived naturally inside your life?

As you write, reflect on:

> What made movement hard to sustain in past seasons

> What assumptions you held about consistency, structure, or "doing it right"

> How real life disrupted those expectations

This is not about blame. It is about understanding what didn't work—and why.

What unspoken rules have shaped your relationship with movement—and which ones are you ready to release?

You might explore:

> Rules about intensity, time, tracking, or sameness

> How those rules affected your willingness to return after disruption

> What principles might feel more supportive than rules

Finish this reflection by writing one or two new movement principles you want to live by.

If movement were designed to live where your life already is, what would it look like in this season?

Consider:

> What forms of movement feel most accessible right now

> What environments or cues could make returning easier

> How you might lower the bar without losing connection

There is no ideal answer—only a livable one.

Chapter 3 — Body Image & Self-Acceptance

Body image is often misunderstood as a surface issue—something about mirrors, clothing sizes, or photographs. But at its core, body image is not about how the body looks. It is about how safe, valued, and at home we feel inside our own skin.

A person can like how they look and still feel deeply disconnected from their body. Another can struggle with appearance and yet feel grounded, present, and at peace. This is because body image is not cosmetic. It is relational.

It reflects whether the body feels like a place we inhabit—or a place we monitor.

Many of us were taught to evaluate our bodies long before we were taught to inhabit them. We learned to scan, critique, compare, and correct. We learned to look at our bodies rather than listen to them. Over time, this creates distance—not just from appearance, but from presence.

When the body becomes an object of observation instead of a partner in experience, self-acceptance becomes difficult. We live just outside ourselves, managing perception rather than participating in life.

Healing body image is less about changing the body and more about changing the story we tell ourselves about it.

How Surveillance Replaced Presence

For many people, body awareness began as body surveillance.

We learned early to notice how we looked sitting, standing, eating, and moving. We learned which parts were acceptable and which needed fixing. This awareness was often praised as responsibility or self-control, even when it came at the cost of ease.

But constant monitoring does not create care.

It creates tension.

The nervous system cannot relax when it is always being watched—even by ourselves. Over time, the body learns that visibility equals evaluation, and presence begins to feel unsafe.

This is why body image struggles are often accompanied by anxiety, dissociation, or exhaustion. The body is not only being lived in. It is being managed.

Reclaiming body image begins with reclaiming presence.

How the Story Shifts Over Time

Body image is not static. It evolves with age, life events, health changes, and the roles we inhabit. What felt tolerable in one season may feel tender in another. What once passed as confidence may later reveal itself as coping.

Many of our earliest beliefs about bodies were inherited rather than chosen. They came from family conversations, cultural expectations, media messages, and unspoken rules about worth. Long before we had language for discernment, we absorbed ideas about what bodies should look like, how they should behave, and what they were allowed to take up.

These messages did not arrive neutrally. They arrived wrapped in a sense of belonging, approval, or protection. Letting them go can feel risky—not because they are true, but because they are familiar.

There were seasons when my body felt like an enemy—especially during times of stress, injury, or change. In those moments, it was easy to reduce my body to a list of problems to solve. My attention narrowed. Compassion thinned.

Over time, something softened. Criticism slowly gave way to curiosity. I began to see my body not as a failure, but as a witness—one that had carried me through every chapter of my life.

That shift did not happen all at once.

It happened through awareness, repetition, and gentleness.

The Difference Between Acceptance and Giving Up

Self-acceptance is often misunderstood as resignation.

But acceptance is not passivity. It is honesty without hostility. It is the decision to stop fighting reality so that energy can be used for care instead of control.

Acceptance does not say, "Nothing can change."

It says, "I will not harm myself in the process of change."

This distinction matters. Many people resist self-acceptance because they fear it will stall progress. In reality, it often does the opposite. When the body is no longer treated as an adversary, cooperation becomes possible.

Peace is not the absence of desire.

It is the absence of war.

Worth That Is Not Tied to Appearance

Confidence rooted in appearance is fragile. It rises and falls with circumstances we cannot control—aging, illness, stress, seasons of life. Confidence rooted in appearance requires constant reinforcement and collapses easily under pressure.

Confidence rooted in worth is steadier.

It grows quietly from how we care for ourselves, how we speak to ourselves, and how we show up in our own lives. It does not depend on mirrors for validation. It does not disappear when the body changes.

What helps me feel confident now is not chasing an image, but remembering a truth: *my worth was never dependent on my appearance.* When I nourish my body well, move gently, and rest without guilt, confidence grows naturally. It feels less like trying to convince myself and more like remembering something I already knew but forgot.

Presence has become more powerful than affirmation.

Being in my body—rather than standing outside it, judging—has done more to heal my body image than any mirror mantra ever did.

Embodiment as Healing

Embodiment is the practice of living from inside the body rather than observing it from the outside.

It is felt through sensation, breath, movement, and stillness. It does not require liking how the body looks. It requires listening to how the body feels.

Embodiment heals body image by shifting the relationship from evaluation to experience.

When you are present in your body—walking, breathing, resting, noticing—there is less mental space for comparison. The body becomes a place you live, not a problem you manage.

This is why gentle movement, mindful breathing, and rest play such a powerful role in healing body image. They return you to yourself without requiring performance.

Stepping Out of Comparison

Comparison is one of the quickest ways to abandon ourselves.

It disconnects us from our own body's history, timing, and needs. It flattens complex stories into surface-level judgments. And it often masquerades as motivation while quietly eroding self-trust.

Comparison thrives in environments of excess input. Too many images. Too many standards. Too much information without integration.

It tends to show up when we are tired, overwhelmed, or emotionally vulnerable. Awareness matters here. When we notice our triggers—certain spaces, images, or internal scripts—we gain the ability to choose differently.

For me, avoiding comparison has meant being intentional about what I consume, both online and internally. When comparison sneaks in, I pause and remind myself that bodies are shaped by different histories, not different worth.

Returning to gratitude for what my body does—rather than what it looks like—helps me return to alignment.

Boundaries are not avoidance.

They are self-respect.

Unlearning Harmful Messages

Many of the most damaging beliefs about our bodies were learned early and reinforced repeatedly. They are not undone through force or shame, but through patience and truth.

Unlearning is an active process.

It requires noticing the old message, naming it gently, and choosing something truer in its place—again and again. This work is repetitive by nature. That does not mean it is failing. It means it is deep.

Criticism may feel familiar, but it does not create change.

Truth does.

I am actively unlearning the belief that my body must be controlled or corrected to be acceptable. I am releasing the idea that rest or softness equals failure. These messages shaped how I moved, how I ate, and how I spoke to myself.

Letting them go has been slow—and deeply freeing.

Healing does not mean never hearing the old voice again.

It means no longer letting it lead.

Meeting Yourself in the Mirror

The mirror often reflects our inner dialogue more than our physical form.

After years of criticism, kindness can feel unfamiliar—almost awkward. Many of us know exactly how to speak harshly to our reflection, but we struggle to speak gently.

This is not a character flaw. It is a learned pattern. Kindness reshapes more than mindset. It creates nervous system safety.

When I look in the mirror now, I try to soften my gaze. Instead of scanning for flaws, I offer gratitude—for endurance, for healing, for presence. Even a simple, "You're doing your best," has begun to change how my body feels to live in.

When the reflection becomes a friend instead of a judge, something profound shifts.

The body relaxes.

Breath deepens.

Defense softens.

Self-Acceptance as Relationship

Self-acceptance is not resignation. It is a relationship. It does not mean loving every part of your body every day. It means choosing not to wage war against it. It means making peace with the body you have in this season, while honoring its story and its wisdom.

Acceptance allows grief without collapse.

> Change without violence.

> Care without condition.

Healing body image is not about arriving at confidence. It is about cultivating compassion. And compassion, practiced consistently, becomes a place where the body can finally relax.

A Different Kind of Peace

Peace does not come from fixing every perceived flaw. It comes from no longer defining yourself by them. This kind of peace is quiet. It does not announce itself. It shows up in small moments—choosing clothes for comfort, resting without apology, moving without self-surveillance.

It is the peace of being at home. And when the body feels like home, self-acceptance stops being a goal and becomes a way of living.

Journal Prompts

When you think about your body, do you experience it more as a place you live—or a place you monitor?

Write about:

> How you tend to relate to your body day to day
>
> Moments when you feel present inside your body
>
> Moments when you notice yourself watching, judging, or managing it

There is no right answer. This is about noticing, not correcting.

What messages about bodies did you learn early—directly or indirectly—and how have they shaped the story you tell about your own?

You may reflect on:

> Family, cultural, or media influences
>
> Ideas about worth, control, or acceptability
>
> Which messages feel true—and which no longer fit

Gently name what you are ready to release, even if you are not ready to fully let it go yet.

What helps you feel most present in your body—not evaluating it, but inhabiting it?

Consider:

> Activities, sensations, or moments that bring you back inside yourself
>
> How your body feels when you are not trying to improve it
>
> What presence offers that comparison never has

Write about how embodiment changes your experience of yourself.

When you encounter your reflection, what tone does your inner voice take—and what would it sound like to soften that voice?

You might explore:

    Familiar patterns of criticism or scanning

    How kindness feels in comparison

    One sentence you could offer yourself that prioritizes safety over approval

This is not about forced affirmation. It is about honest gentleness.

What would it look like to relate to your body as a partner rather than a problem in this season of your life?

Reflect on:

    Where you may be asking your body to earn worth

    Where you might offer care without condition

    How acceptance could coexist with growth, change, or desire

End by completing this sentence in your own words:

    Self-acceptance, for me, looks like…

Chapter 4 — Tracking Progress Beyond the Scale

For many of us, the scale became the loudest voice in the room.

It told us whether we were succeeding or failing, whether we were disciplined or careless, whether our efforts "counted." Over time, it didn't just measure weight—it began to measure worth. A single number could shape the mood of an entire day, even when nothing else had changed. A higher number could undo a week of good choices. A lower number could temporarily quiet self-criticism—even if nothing meaningful had shifted internally.

The scale was treated as objective, neutral, and authoritative. But its influence was anything but neutral. It shaped behavior, self-talk, and emotional safety. It taught many of us to outsource trust in our bodies to an external device.

But the scale has always been limited.

> It measures mass, not meaning.

> It measures gravity, not health.

> It measures weight, not wisdom.

The body communicates progress in ways no number can capture—through energy, mood, regulation, resilience, and the quiet ease of daily living. Healing often shows up there first.

This chapter invites a shift: from external measurement to internal awareness, from judgment to listening, from urgency to trust.

How the Scale Became an Authority

The scale did not become powerful overnight. It earned authority slowly—through repetition, reinforcement, and cultural agreement. It was presented as neutral data, a helpful tool, a motivator. Over time, many of us stopped questioning it. But tools shape behavior. And authority shapes identity.

When the scale is given the final word, it trains us to look outside ourselves for feedback. Hunger becomes suspect. Fatigue becomes inconvenient. Progress is only validated if the number on the scale agrees.

This dynamic disconnects us from the body's internal signals. We stop asking how we feel and start asking what the scale says. And when those two answers conflict, the scale usually wins.

This is not because the scale is evil.

It is because it is loud.

Recognizing Non-Scale Victories

Some of the most meaningful progress happens in small, ordinary moments.

> More consistent energy throughout the day.
>
> Feeling calmer around food or movement.
>
> Less internal negotiation.
>
> Fewer crashes.
>
> More stable moods.
>
> A quieter relationship with choice.

These changes don't show up on a scale, but they profoundly affect the quality of life.

Non-scale victories reflect functional health—health that supports how we live, not just how we look. Often, they appear long before any visible change. Learning to notice and celebrate them reinforces self-trust and motivation far more sustainably than chasing numbers ever could.

The problem is not that these victories don't exist.

It's that we were never taught to look for them.

Acknowledging progress when it isn't easily measured requires a different kind of attentiveness. It asks us to pay attention to how our days feel, how our bodies respond, and how our inner dialogue shifts.

This kind of noticing is subtle. And because it is subtle, it is powerful.

Why Healing Shows Up Internally First

The body prioritizes survival and regulation before appearance.

When care improves—through nourishment, gentler movement, rest, or stress reduction—the nervous system often stabilizes first. Hormones begin to regulate. Inflammation quiets. Digestion improves. Sleep deepens.

These changes may not move the scale immediately, but they are foundational. They create conditions that enable long-term health.

Ignoring these signs because the scale has not changed is like dismissing healing because it is quiet.

Internal repair often precedes visible change.

Redefining Progress

When progress is defined solely by weight loss, everything else is at risk of being dismissed.

Better sleep becomes irrelevant.

Improved mood goes unnoticed.

Increased confidence is overshadowed.

A calmer relationship with food is minimized.

But progress includes habits, mindset, regulation, and awareness. It includes sleeping better, thinking more clearly, and making choices without guilt or urgency. It includes feeling less reactive and more present.

It includes resilience.

Healing is rarely linear. There are pauses, fluctuations, and seasons where internal repair is happening long before anything looks different on the outside. When definitions of success expand, pressure softens. Discouragement loosens its grip.

In this season, progress may look like stability rather than change. And stability matters.

When Stability Is the Victory

Stability doesn't sell well in a culture addicted to transformation.

But stability is often the greatest gift the body can offer after years of stress, dieting, or overexertion. It means the system is no longer constantly compensating.

> Stable energy.
>
> Stable mood.
>
> Stable digestion.
>
> Stable appetite.

These are not plateaus.

> They are repairs.

Learning to honor stability as progress is one of the most radical shifts a person can make. It requires patience. It requires trust. It requires letting go of urgency. And it allows the body to exhale.

What Success Feels Like

Success is often quieter than we expect. It feels like ease. Like cooperation instead of resistance. Like a body that is less tense, less inflamed, less braced against itself. It feels like balance—physically and mentally. When success is defined by sensation rather than strain, the body becomes a source of feedback instead of fear.

Learning to notice these sensations builds body trust. When we tune in, the body offers information: fewer aches, steadier energy, smoother transitions between effort and rest. These are signs of alignment.

While they may not impress an algorithm, they do sustain a life.

Listening to Functional Signals

The body often improves function before appearance changes.

> Energy steadies.

> Digestion becomes more predictable.

> Mood evens out.

> Skin reflects internal balance.

> Sleep deepens.

> Cravings soften.

These systems respond quickly when the body feels supported—even if weight remains unchanged for a time.

Tracking patterns—not obsessively, but gently—can offer insight without judgment. Noticing how food, rest, stress, and movement affect these systems builds awareness without turning the body back into a project.

This kind of tracking asks different questions:

- How do I feel after eating this way?
- How does my energy respond to rest?
- What happens when stress decreases?
- When do I feel most regulated?

These shifts influence daily life in tangible ways. When energy is steadier and digestion calmer, decisions feel easier. Life feels more manageable. That matters.

Awareness Without Surveillance

There is a difference between awareness and surveillance.

> Awareness listens.

> Surveillance evaluates.

The scale encourages surveillance. It reduces complexity to a single metric. Awareness expands understanding.

Releasing the scale does not mean abandoning awareness. It means choosing a wiser form—one that respects nuance and context. You are allowed to notice patterns without punishing yourself for them.

When the Scale Stalls

Plateaus are a normal part of long-term health change.

> They are not a verdict.

> They are not a failure.

> They are not proof that nothing is working.

But emotionally, they can feel heavy. When the scale doesn't move, frustration, doubt, and discouragement often surface. These feelings deserve compassion, not correction. Fighting them usually intensifies them. Redirecting focus back to internal markers—energy, mood, regulation—can ground us again. It reminds us that healing is still happening, even when the scale is quiet.

Motivation grows when goals are internal rather than external. Remembering why you began—peace, vitality, sustainability—anchors commitment when numbers fluctuate.

Healing is not a race. It unfolds on the body's timeline, not our impatience.

Letting Go Without Losing Control

One of the biggest fears around releasing the scale is losing accountability. But accountability does not require punishment. It requires honesty.

Internal accountability asks: "How am I actually doing?"

External accountability asks: "What does the number say?"

The first builds self-trust.

The second often undermines it.

Letting go of the scale is not about pretending numbers don't exist. It is about refusing to let them define reality. You are allowed to choose the information that helps you care for yourself.

Trusting a Bigger Picture

The scale tells a very small story.

Your body is telling a much larger one—through how you feel, how you function, and how you live. Learning to listen to that story requires patience and presence, but it leads to a deeper, steadier kind of progress.

Releasing the scale doesn't mean abandoning awareness.

It means choosing a wiser one. And when progress is measured by wholeness rather than weight, the body is finally allowed to heal without being rushed.

I still weigh myself every day, but I realize there are natural fluctuations that happen throughout the day and the week. So, I average the daily measurements each week, which allows me to look for trends rather than being controlled by a single daily number. Some people cannot do this, and that is okay, too.

A Quieter Kind of Success

Success does not always look dramatic.

Sometimes it looks like fewer internal battles.

Sometimes it looks like steadier days.

Sometimes it looks like peace where there used to be pressure.

These changes may never be reflected in a number.

But they will be reflected in your life, and that is the kind of progress worth tracking.

Journal Prompts

What role has the scale played in shaping how you evaluate progress, effort, or worth?

Write about:

How a number has influenced your mood or self-talk

What you learned to believe when the number went up or down

Whether the scale felt neutral or authoritative

This is not about judgment. It is about understanding influence.

What changes have you noticed in your body or life that no number could capture?

You might reflect on:

Energy, mood, sleep, digestion, focus, or calm

How daily choices feel now compared to before

Subtle shifts that made life easier or steadier

Name at least one change that mattered—even if it never showed up on a scale.

If progress were measured by how your body feels rather than how it weighs, what would you notice?

Consider:

Sensations of ease or tension

How your body responds to food, rest, or movement

When your system feels most regulated

Write without trying to rank or improve—only observe.

Where has stability shown up in your life—and how have you responded to it?

Reflect on:

> Periods where things felt steadier rather than "changing"
>
> Whether you've dismissed stability as "not enough"
>
> How honoring steadiness might support long-term healing

Complete this sentence in your own words:

> Stability is meaningful because…

How does awareness feel different in your body than surveillance?

You may explore:

> How your body responds when it is listened to rather than evaluated
>
> The difference between noticing patterns and policing behavior
>
> What kind of awareness feels supportive rather than stressful

Let this be an honest comparison, not a conclusion.

What does success feel like in your body—not on paper, not in numbers, but in lived experience?

Describe:

> How success shows up physically or emotionally
>
> What feels quieter, softer, or less effortful now
>
> How your definition of progress may be expanding

There is no need to impress anyone here—not even yourself.

What fears surface when you imagine releasing the scale—and what truths might gently meet those fears?

Write about:

      What you worry you might lose

      What you might gain in peace or clarity

      How internal accountability could look in this season

Fear does not mean you are wrong. It means something important is changing.

Chapter 5 — Identity & Health Transformation

Health transformation is never just physical.

Long before the body changes in visible ways, something quieter begins to shift internally: beliefs soften, awareness deepens, and old narratives loosen their grip. The internal landscape begins to rearrange itself. And with those changes comes something many people don't expect: a shift in identity.

Sometimes that shift feels gentle, almost imperceptible.

Sometimes it feels disorienting, even unsettling.

This chapter invites reflection not on who you are trying to become, but on who you are returning to. True transformation is not about constructing a new self from scratch. It is about aligning with the truest one—the one that has been there all along, waiting not for correction, but for support.

Identity change is rarely announced. It happens quietly, through repetition, through choice, through moments where you respond differently than you once did. Over time, those moments accumulate, and the story you tell about yourself begins to change.

When Self-Image Begins to Shift

Self-image often changes before we consciously notice it changing. At first, the shift is subtle.

It shows up in language.

A softer inner voice.

Less urgency to fix.

More curiosity where criticism once lived.

Beliefs that once felt unquestionable begin to loosen, not because they were argued against, but because they no longer fit.

Physical changes may lag behind, but internally, something has already moved.

For me, one of the most significant shifts was releasing the belief that I was undisciplined. That label followed me for a long time. It shaped how I interpreted my struggles and how harshly I spoke to myself. Every difficulty became evidence. Every inconsistency only reinforced the story.

But as my relationship with my body changed, so did my interpretation of my past. I began to see something different. I wasn't undisciplined—I was carrying a great deal.

Stress.

Trauma.

Expectations.

Survival patterns that required constant effort.

When I stopped fighting my body and started caring for it, respect replaced criticism. Not because I became someone new, but because I finally saw myself clearly. That clarity did not arrive all at once. It arrived through awareness, repetition, and gentleness.

Grief as Part of Growth

Growth often includes grief.

Grief for old versions of ourselves.

Grief for the years spent believing something untrue.

Grief for how hard we were on ourselves when we didn't yet know another way.

This grief is not self-indulgent. It is honest.

Maturity includes the ability to look back without contempt. To recognize that earlier versions of us were doing the best they could with the tools they had. To hold regret without self-punishment.

Honoring that grief is part of integration. It allows us to move forward without pretending the past didn't matter.

A transformation that skips grief tends to recreate the same patterns under new names. A transformation that honors grief creates room for compassion—and compassion changes how identity is carried forward.

Identity Is Built in Repetition, Not Revelation

Identity is not formed in declarations. It is formed in patterns. The choices we repeat—how we eat, move, rest, and respond—quietly shape who we become. This process is ongoing. There is no finished version waiting at the end, no moment when the work is complete, and our identity is locked in place.

As my lifestyle changed, so did my sense of self. Not dramatically. Gradually. I noticed more patience. More discernment. Less urgency to prove anything. Listening—rather than pushing—became a defining trait. Not because it sounded virtuous, but because it worked.

An identity rooted in alignment feels steadier than one rooted in outcomes. When worth is no longer tied to results, the nervous system relaxes. Decisions feel cleaner. Life feels less performative.

Becoming is not about striving forward into something artificial. It is about settling into what feels true.

The Difference Between Identity and Performance

Many identities are reinforced through performance.

Being "the disciplined one."

Being "the strong one."

Being "the one who never quits."

These identities often look admirable from the outside. But internally, they can be exhausting. Performance-based identity requires constant maintenance. It depends on consistency that ignores context and effort that overrides need.

When health is tied to performance, rest feels like failure. Flexibility feels like weakness. Adaptation feels like regression.

But an identity that is rooted in alignment feels different. It does not require constant proving. It allows change without collapse. It recognizes that who you are is not dependent on what you produce. This shift—from performance to alignment—is one of the most stabilizing aspects of health transformation.

Releasing Identities Built for Survival

Not every identity we've held was chosen freely.

Some were formed to survive.

Pushing through exhaustion.

Ignoring signals.

Being "the reliable one."

Being the one who never rests.

Being the one who keeps going no matter the cost.

These identities often served a real purpose. They helped us cope when resources were limited and safety felt uncertain. They kept life functioning when pausing was not an option. Letting go of them can feel like losing a familiar role. There may be fear underneath the release—fear of becoming unrecognizable, of disappointing others, of losing worth.

Part of my own transition has been recognizing that earlier versions of me were doing their best with what they had. Honoring them—without continuing the patterns they relied on—has been deeply healing.

Awareness creates choice. It allows us to thank what once helped us survive, and still choose differently now. Release does not require shame. It requires compassion.

When the Body Signals That Identity Is Changing

As identity shifts, the body's needs often shift too. What once felt supportive may begin to feel demanding. What once felt productive may begin to feel depleting. This can be confusing, especially if old identities were reinforced by intensity or endurance.

Healing asks us to update our approach—not out of fear, but out of respect.

Listening replaces control as the guiding principle.

Right now, my body responds best to consistency and patience. Gentle movement. Intentional nourishment. Rest without guilt. I am learning that support does not have to be intense to be effective.

Boundaries have become part of care. Protecting healing sometimes means doing less, not more. That choice reflects growth, not regression. When identity shifts from proving to partnering, the body no longer has to escalate its signals to be heard.

Boundaries as Evidence of Maturity

Early in many health journeys, boundaries feel restrictive. It is usually later that they feel protective.

Saying no to certain demands—physical, emotional, relational—is not a sign of fragility. It is a sign that the body's wisdom is being respected. Boundaries preserve energy. They support regulation. They allow healing to continue rather than unravel.

Identity matures when boundaries are no longer experienced as punishment, but as stewardship.

Living From Truth, Not Just Believing It

Transformation deepens when truth moves from concept to practice. Many of us believe we are worthy of care, but we live as if that worth must still be earned. We agree with the idea intellectually, while our daily choices tell a different story.

Embodied truth reshapes decisions.

It changes self-talk.

It influences what we tolerate, what we pursue, and what we release.

One truth I am learning to live from is this:

I am worthy of care now.

Not later.

Not after I arrive somewhere else.

Right here, right now.

That truth changes everything from how I eat to how I move to how I rest. Knowing that I am worthy of and deserve care right now changes how I respond to my own needs. It has become a foundation rather than a thought.

Alignment does not happen all at once. It happens through daily practice—through choosing trust over fear, again and again.

Identity as a Place to Stand

When identity is rooted in truth rather than aspiration, health becomes more stable. There is less urgency. Less self-surveillance. Less pressure to become something else.

The body no longer has to argue for care.

Care is already included.

This is where transformation becomes sustainable—not because everything is perfect, but because the relationship is intact.

Honoring Who You Have Been, Stepping Into Who You Are

Identity transformation is not about erasing the past. It is about integrating it. It's about honoring who you have been, recognizing who you are becoming, and supporting your body as a partner in the process rather than a project to manage.

Health becomes sustainable when it is rooted in identity—not aspiration. And when identity is grounded in truth, the body no longer has to fight to be heard. It can finally participate fully in the life you are building.

Journal Prompts

When you reflect on your health journey, who do you feel you are returning to rather than trying to become?

Write about:

> Qualities you had before criticism or pressure shaped you

> Traits that feel natural rather than forced

> Parts of you that feel familiar in a grounding way

Transformation may be less about construction and more about remembering.

How has your inner dialogue changed over time?

Notice:

> Is your tone softer?

> Are you less urgent?

> Do you respond differently to setbacks?

Write specific phrases your inner voice used to say — and what it says now.

What do you grieve about earlier seasons of your life or health journey?

You might explore:

> Years spent believing something untrue

> Ways you pushed yourself beyond your limits

> Identities you held for survival

Now write:

"That version of me was doing the best she could with…"

Allow grief and compassion to coexist.

Where in your life does performance still show up?

Where do you feel:

The need to prove

The need to maintain an image

The pressure to be consistent regardless of context

Now ask:

What would alignment look like instead?

What repeated choices (patterns) are quietly shaping your new identity?

Small examples count:

Choosing rest

Lowering the bar on hard days

Listening before reacting

Eating with presence

Identity is not declared. It is practiced. List the patterns you are repeating now.

Where have you set boundaries that reflect maturity rather than limitation?

Write about:

A boundary that once felt restrictive but now feels protective

A "no" that preserved your energy

A change in how you relate to your body's limits

Boundaries are evidence of identity shifting toward stewardship.

Chapter 6 — Rebuilding Trust with Your Body

Body trust is rarely lost all at once.

It erodes slowly—through years of ignoring signals, overriding needs, and absorbing messages that the body cannot be trusted. Many of us were taught, subtly or explicitly, that hunger should be controlled, pain should be pushed through, and rest should be earned. Over time, listening felt risky. Control felt safer.

Disconnection often begins as protection. Stress, trauma, dieting, illness, and survival demands can interrupt body awareness. In those seasons, tuning out may have been the only way to keep going. That disconnection was not failure—it was adaptation.

Noticing it now is not cause for shame. It is the first step toward reconnection.

When Disconnection Made Sense

There were seasons in my life when I lived far from my body. I pushed past exhaustion. I ignored hunger and rest. I treated discomfort as something to overcome rather than understand. I believed that responding to my body's needs would slow me down, weaken me, or make life harder.

At the time, that distance felt necessary. Life required endurance. Responsibilities did not pause just because my body was struggling. Looking back, I can see that disconnection wasn't a lack of discipline—it was a form of self-protection. My body carried me through those seasons in the only way it knew how.

Disconnection is often misunderstood as neglect. In reality, it is frequently a survival strategy. When listening feels overwhelming or unsafe, the nervous system learns to mute sensation. This is not a conscious choice. It is an intelligent response to prolonged stress.

Rebuilding trust does not begin by judging those past choices. It begins by honoring the context in which they were made.

Why Control Feels Safer Than Listening

Control offers *predictability*. Rules feel clear. Structure feels stabilizing. External systems promise certainty when internal cues feel unreliable or frightening. Many people learn to trust plans, metrics, or schedules long before they trust sensation.

Listening, by contrast, feels ambiguous.

> Signals change.

> Needs vary.

> Rest and hunger do not follow neat formulas.

When worth is tied to productivity or restraint, listening can feel like a loss of control rather than a source of wisdom.

For a long time, I believed that discipline meant overriding my body. That strength meant not needing anything. That responding to discomfort was indulgent. Those beliefs didn't come from nowhere. They were reinforced by culture, expectations, and environments that did not reward slowing down.

Control kept me functional. I wasn't even aware of the power of listening to my body. Understanding this has been essential. Trust cannot be rebuilt if we shame ourselves for not having actually listened in the first place.

How Trust Is Actually Rebuilt

Trust is not restored through force or perfection. It is rebuilt through follow-through. Trust grows when signals are met with response—not instantly, not perfectly, but consistently enough that the body learns it is safe to communicate again. This looks like resting when tired, eating when hungry, and stopping when something doesn't feel right.

These choices may seem ordinary. They are not. They are foundational. Gentle consistency matters more than intensity. Predictability matters more than performance. When care is reliable, the nervous system relaxes, and when the nervous system relaxes, the body speaks more clearly.

Safety invites communication. Every time you respond with care instead of criticism, trust grows. Every time you pause instead of pushing, the body learns that it no longer has to escalate its signals to be heard.

Trust Is Built in Small Moments

Rebuilding trust does not require a dramatic change.

It happens in small moments:

- choosing to rest before collapse
- noticing hunger without moralizing it
- stopping movement when pain *begins* instead of *after injury*
- adjusting plans instead of forcing compliance

These moments are easy to overlook, but to the body, they matter deeply.

Trust is built through reliability and showing up again and again with respect. This is why perfection is not only unnecessary—it is counterproductive. Missed cues do not destroy trust. What matters is returning to listening when you notice you've drifted. Trust grows through repair, not flawless execution.

Learning the Body's Language Again

The body speaks constantly—through sensation, emotion, and energy. After long periods of disconnection, those signals may feel muted, overwhelming, or confusing. This does not mean the body is broken. It means the channel has been quiet for a long time.

Curiosity helps decode the language.

Instead of asking, "What's wrong with me?"

The question becomes, "What might this be pointing to?"

For me, the body often speaks through subtle shifts:

- tension in the jaw or shoulders
- a sense of restlessness
- irritability without obvious cause
- fatigue that feels heavier than usual

These are not inconveniences. What they are is information, and information is power. Pausing to notice patterns—rather than reacting immediately—has changed the way I live in my body. When I stay present long enough to listen, the message usually clarifies. Listening does not mean obeying every impulse. It means staying attentive long enough to understand what the body is trying to communicate.

The Role of Emotion in Body Trust

Emotions are part of the body's language. Many people were taught to separate their emotions from their physical experience. In reality, they are deeply connected. Emotional shifts often signal unmet needs—rest, safety, nourishment, crossed boundaries. When emotional signals are ignored, the body often compensates through physical symptoms. Fatigue. Pain. Tension. Discomfort.

Rebuilding trust includes allowing emotion to be information rather than an unpleasant interruption. This does not mean indulging every feeling. It means acknowledging emotion as part of the feedback system rather than something to suppress or fix.

What Made Trust Difficult

Many of us were taught to replace internal wisdom with external rules. Diet culture, perfectionism, comparison, and shame all disrupt listening. They train their attention outward rather than inward. They reward control rather than responsiveness.

When worth is tied to restraint or performance, trusting the body feels dangerous. Hunger becomes suspect. Fatigue feels like weakness. Pain feels like failure.

I absorbed the message that my body needed strict control to be acceptable. That left little room for curiosity or compassion. Releasing that belief has been challenging. It has also been liberating. Trust does not mean the body will never struggle. It means the struggle is met with care rather than punishment.

From Control to Cooperation

Before a partnership with your body can be established, there needs to be cooperation. This stage matters. Cooperation looks like compromise instead of domination. It acknowledges both needs and limits. It allows structure without rigidity.

For me, cooperation meant adjusting expectations rather than abandoning them. Choosing gentler forms of movement. Eating in ways that felt supportive instead of restrictive. Allowing rest without negotiating its worth. Cooperation is where trust begins to stabilize.

From Cooperation to Partnership

The most profound shift happens when the body is no longer treated as a problem to fix.

Allies are listened to, not battled.

Partnership invites collaboration instead of control. When the body is viewed as an ally, motivation changes. Self-talk softens. Care replaces correction.

For me, this required changing the question entirely.

Not, "What's wrong with you?"

But, "How can I support you?"

That single shift significantly changed how I thought about and interacted with my body. Movement became care rather than compliance. Food became nourishment rather than negotiation. Rest became wisdom rather than weakness.

Partnership isn't about indulgence; it's about alignment.

Trust as a Daily Practice

Rebuilding body trust is not a single decision, made once and done. It is a practice. It grows through small acts of respect that are repeated over time. Through choosing partnership when control feels tempting. Through listening even when the message is inconvenient.

Some days, listening confirms what you hoped to hear. Other days, it asks for change. Trust grows when both are honored. As trust rebuilds, the body responds—not by becoming perfect, but by becoming more cooperative, more communicative, more at ease. Signals soften. Recovery improves. Resistance decreases. The body no longer has to shout to be heard.

When Trust Feels Fragile Again

There will be days when trust feels harder. Stress returns. Old habits resurface. Control feels tempting. This does not mean trust has failed. It means life has shifted.

Trust isn't lost through struggle; it is built back through repair. Resuming listening—even after mistakes—supports safety much more effectively than self-criticism.

Allowing Healing to Unfold

When the body feels safe enough to be heard, healing no longer has to be forced. It can unfold at the pace trust allows. This pace may feel slower than ambition prefers, but it is often faster than burnout permits.

Rebuilding trust does not guarantee comfort. It guarantees a relationship, and that relationship is what allows the body to heal without fear.

Journal Prompts

When in your life did disconnecting from your body feel necessary?

Write about:

> Seasons when listening felt unsafe or overwhelming

> Times you pushed through exhaustion, hunger, or pain

> What that disconnection protected you from

End with:

> "At that time, my body and I were doing our best to…"

This is not about blame. It is about context.

Where does control still feel safer than listening?

Notice:

> Do you rely more on rules than sensation?

> Do you override fatigue to "stay disciplined"?

> Does hunger make you uneasy?

Now ask:

What am I afraid might happen if I listened instead?

Explore that fear gently.

What is one recent moment when you responded to your body with care instead of correction?

It might have been:

> Resting sooner

> Eating without guilt

> Adjusting movement

Pausing when overwhelmed

Write about how that moment felt.

Even small repairs rebuild trust.

Complete these two reflections:

"When I treat my body like a problem, I tend to…"

"When I treat my body like a partner, I tend to…"

What shifts in your tone? In your posture? In your decisions?

Partnership begins with how you ask the question.

If rebuilding body trust were your priority this week, what would change in how you respond to your needs?

Consider:

Hunger

Fatigue

Emotional signals

Physical discomfort

Write one commitment in this format:

"When my body signals _____, I will respond with _____."

Keep it simple. Keep it realistic.

Trust grows through follow-through.

Chapter 7 — Loving Your Body Through Movement

There is a profound difference between moving in your body and moving with it.

For many of us, movement has been framed as an obligation—something we do because we should, because we're behind, because something needs fixing. Even when intentions are good, that posture quietly reinforces distance. The body becomes a task rather than a companion. Movement becomes corrective instead of connective.

But movement can be an expression of love.

When movement is guided by reverence instead of demand, it becomes a language of care. It communicates gratitude rather than correction. Presence rather than pressure. This chapter invites a reimagining of movement—not as something required of you, but as something offered to your body.

When Movement Carries a History

Movement rarely arrives in the present moment empty-handed. It carries memory. Conditioning. Emotion. For many people, movement is tied to judgment, metrics, comparison, or punishment—even if no one explicitly called it that. The body remembers being pushed, evaluated, measured, and corrected. It remembers when movement was used to override hunger, exhaustion, or grief. This is why simply "changing your mindset" around movement rarely works.

The body does not respond to slogans. It responds to experience. Loving movement must be felt in the body, not declared by the mind. It must be demonstrated through consistency, respect, and attunement. Only then does the nervous system begin to relax its guard.

When Movement Becomes Attentive

Loving movement feels different in the body. It feels attuned and responsive It feels gentle without being passive and strong without being harsh. It supports rather than coerces. It leaves the body feeling heard rather than judged. Attentive movement listens before it acts.

Instead of asking, "What should I do today?"

The question becomes, "What does my body need support with today?"

For me, acts of love in movement look like listening closely—choosing gentle strength when stability is needed, walking when grounding feels supportive, and stretching when tension asks for release. The intention matters as much as the motion. When movement feels attentive rather than demanding, it becomes restorative rather than depleting. Care-based movement builds trust because it respects limits instead of testing them.

Love Does Not Rush the Body

One of the clearest signs that movement is rooted in love is pace. Love does not rush. It does not demand immediacy. It does not panic at slowness.

Many people associate slow movement with failure or regression. In reality, slowness often allows the body to reorganize more intelligently. It gives space for coordination, breath, and sensation to work together.

When I move slowly, I notice things I used to miss—how my weight shifts, where I brace unnecessarily, where I'm holding tension out of habit rather than need. Slowing down has revealed not weakness, but information.

Love gives the body time to speak.

Celebrating the Body You Have Today

Love notices capability. Celebration shifts focus from what is missing to what is present. It honors ability without comparison and without denial of loss.

Bodies change over time. Seasons that we pass through during the course of our lives alter our body's capacity. Some abilities grow. Others recede. Loving the body means acknowledging all of it honestly.

Celebration does not require pretending everything is fine. It requires noticing what is here.

I've learned to celebrate by noticing what feels easier—standing longer, breathing deeper, moving with less pain, recovering more quickly…and yes, even that my cheeks no longer jiggle when I walk. These moments might seem small, but they are meaningful. They reflect adaptation, resilience, and care.

Gratitude strengthens connection. It brings us into a relationship with the body we inhabit now—not the one we remember or imagine.

Grief and Love Can Coexist

Loving your body does not mean denying grief.

There are losses that deserve acknowledgment—movements you once loved, capacities that no longer feel available, rhythms that have changed. Ignoring that grief does not protect the body. It isolates it.

Love allows grief without letting it become contempt.

I have learned to hold both: gratitude for what my body can do and tenderness for what has changed. That balance keeps movement honest. It prevents denial on one side and resentment on the other.

Love tells the truth kindly.

Movement as a Sacred Act

Worship does not require words. It can be embodied, lived, and offered through presence. Movement becomes sacred when it is done with awareness and gratitude—when attention is placed not on performance but on participation. Ordinary motion—walking, breathing, stretching—becomes meaningful when intention aligns.

For me, walking outdoors feels like worship. Breathing deeply. Noticing light, air, rhythm, and the environment around me. Moving in step with the day rather than racing against it. In those moments, movement feels like an offering instead of a task.

Presence transforms motion into prayer. Sacred movement does not require special space or time. It requires attention. It happens when the body is allowed to move as it is, without being measured, restrained, or compared.

When Movement Is About Belonging

One of the quiet gifts of loving movement is belonging.

When movement is no longer about earning worth, the body becomes a place you want to inhabit rather than escape from. You begin to feel at home in motion—not evaluated, not monitored, just present.

This sense of belonging is deeply regulating to the nervous system. It reduces hypervigilance. It softens internal pressure. It creates safety where effort once lived. The body does not thrive under scrutiny. It thrives under care.

Releasing What No Longer Serves

Love also discerns.

Growth requires releasing movement patterns that no longer align with the body's needs. What once felt empowering may later feel depleting. Letting go is not regression—it is wisdom.

There are forms of high-intensity or rigid routines that no longer serve me in this season. Releasing them was uncomfortable at first. Old beliefs surfaced—about discipline, worth, and effort. But my body responded with relief, and letting go revealed something important:

> Much of what I believed was strength was actually bracing.

When movement is guided by love, discernment replaces guilt. Space opens for practices that support who you are now, not who you once had to be.

The Myth That Love Is Soft

Loving movement is often misunderstood as indulgent or weak. In truth, it requires discernment, restraint, and trust. It asks us to resist urgency, tolerate ambiguity, and stay present rather than chase reassurance through intensity. This is not passive. It is deeply intentional.

Supportive strength feels expansive rather than restrictive. It allows breath. It allows adjustment. It allows recovery. Bracing feels rigid, urgent, and fear-driven. Love feels steady. Learning the difference has changed how I move—and how I live.

How Love Changes Motivation

Fear-based movement relies on pressure.

Love-based movement relies on the relationship.

When movement is motivated by fear—fear of decline, fear of weight gain, fear of judgment—it is fragile. It collapses under stress. When life gets hard, fear drains energy instead of providing it.

When movement is motivated by love, it becomes steadier. Not because motivation is constant, but because the relationship remains.

I return to movement now, not because I'm afraid of what will happen if I don't— but because I value how my body feels when I care for it. That shift in how I view moving my body changes everything about how I show up for my body.

After Movement: Listening to the Aftertaste

One of the most revealing questions after movement is not, "How hard was it?" but "How do I feel afterward?"

Care-based movement leaves a different aftertaste:

- more connection

- more calm
- more appreciation
- less judgment

The body remembers how it was treated.

When movement strengthens partnership rather than muscles alone, the body becomes a place we feel at home in. Loving movement does not ask how much was done. It asks how the body was treated.

Love as the Measure

In a culture obsessed with metrics, love offers a different measure.

Not distance.

Not duration.

Not intensity.

But respect.

Did the movement support the body today?

Did it honor limits?

Did it leave the body feeling safer versus threatened?

When the answer is yes, something essential has been accomplished—whether or not it looks impressive from the outside.

An Ongoing Invitation

Loving your body through movement is not a destination. It is a posture you return to—again and again—especially when old habits try to reassert themselves. Some days love looks like movement. Other days it looks like rest. Both can be acts of care.

When the body is honored rather than pushed, it responds—not with perfection, but with trust. And trust is what allows movement to remain part of life—not as an obligation, but as a relationship.

Journal Prompts

When did movement stop feeling joyful and start feeling required?

Reflect on:

What messages shaped your relationship with movement?

Was movement ever tied to fixing, proving, or earning?

What emotions tend to surface when you think about exercise now?

Finish this sentence:

"Movement began to feel heavy when…"

How do you know when you are moving at your body instead of with it?

Notice:

What does your inner voice sound like in those moments?

What happens to your breath, pace, or posture?

What feels different afterward?

Now imagine:

If I moved with my body today, it might look like…

What type of movement currently feels most supportive to your nervous system?

Describe:

How your body feels during it

How your body feels after it

What makes it feel safe or connective

Then write:

"Loving movement, for me, feels like…"

Is there a form of movement you miss?

Allow space for:

    Grief over what has changed

    Tenderness toward your body's current limits

Now gently balance it:

        "Today, I am grateful my body can still…"

Love holds both loss and appreciation.

After your next movement session, reflect on this question:

    How did my body feel afterward — physically, emotionally, and mentally?

Use these cues:

    Did I feel calmer or more braced?

    More connected or more critical?

    Supported or depleted?

Then complete:

        "Today's movement honored my body because…"

Let love—not intensity—be the measure.

Chapter 8 — Posture, Alignment & Pain Prevention

Posture is often reduced to instruction: sit up straight, pull your shoulders back, don't slouch. I remember distinctly many times when my mother would instruct me to sit up straight and stop slouching. The times my sisters and I were instructed to walk across the room with a book balanced on our heads to teach us to walk tall and upright, to glide rather than strut or worse…STOMP across the room. That was fun. My sisters and I made it into a game.

But posture is not a moral failing or a discipline problem. It is a language.

How we sit, stand, and move reflects how we carry ourselves through life—how safe we feel, how alert we are, how much pressure we are holding, and how much permission we give ourselves to take up space. Alignment shapes breath, mood, confidence, and pain levels, often in quiet ways that go unnoticed until discomfort demands attention. This chapter is not about achieving "perfect posture." It is about learning to listen to how your body is holding your life.

Posture as a Record of Experience

The body keeps a record long after the mind has moved on. Posture reflects not only habits, but history. It carries the imprint of years spent adapting—leaning forward to stay alert, collapsing inward to feel smaller, bracing to stay prepared. These shapes are not flaws. They are strategies.

Many of us learned early that being relaxed was not safe. That staying alert mattered more than being comfortable. That carrying responsibility required holding tension. Over time, those adaptations became posture. This is why posture cannot be corrected through command alone. The body does not respond to orders. It responds to safety.

Where the Body Holds What the Mind Carries

Most tension is not random. It gathers in familiar places. For many people, it settles in the shoulders, jaw, neck, hips, or lower back. These are not weaknesses; they are load-bearing areas—physically and emotionally. Stress, concentration, vigilance, grief, and responsibility all have postural expressions.

> The shoulders often carry obligation.

> The jaw holds restraint and unspoken words.

> The hips absorb instability and vigilance.

> The lower back braces under pressure.

I notice tension collecting most reliably in my shoulders and jaw, especially during focused or stressful moments. The body tightens not because it is malfunctioning, but because it is bracing.

When I pause long enough to notice, the message is rarely "push through." It is more often an invitation to breathe, soften, shift position, or release effort that is no longer needed.

Awareness changes everything here. Tension that is noticed early can be addressed gently. Tension that is ignored often escalates into pain.

Why "Fix Your Posture" Often Fails

Traditional posture advice assumes the body is lazy. In reality, the body is adaptive.

When someone tells you to "sit up straight," what they're often asking is for more muscular effort. But effort is rarely what's missing. Support is.

Forcing posture without support creates:

- increased muscle fatigue
- shallow breathing
- more bracing
- greater pain over time

The body resists being commanded when it feels unsafe. It compensates when alignment feels like a strain rather than supportive. Posture is not something we hold. It is something we return to.

As a side note, there is a field of study typically referred to as Body Language, aka Kinesics. Kinesics is a fancy academic term for the study of nonverbal communication, especially body movement—posture, gestures, facial expressions, eye contact, and how people use space when they interact. I have been a people watcher as long as I can remember, mostly alert in my environment to predict the behavior of people who were, to say the least, volatile. One thing that slumped posture reveals is often an unconscious desire to protect our soft, vulnerable parts from harm. It is a fascinating field of study.

However, that is not what I am speaking to in this chapter. In this chapter, I am speaking to something more intimate — not what posture signals to the world, but what it reveals about how safe you feel inside your own body and how your nervous system organizes itself in response.

Alignment as Support, Not Control

Alignment works best when it feels cooperative. Small habits shape posture far more than dramatic corrections. Gentle cues invite alignment without rigidity. They respect the body's design instead of fighting it.

Supportive alignment feels like:

- weight evenly distributed through the feet
- the spine stacked rather than stiffened
- shoulders resting instead of pulled back
- breath moving freely through the ribs

These are not positions to maintain. They are references to return to. Over time, repetition teaches the nervous system safety. Alignment becomes easier not because we're trying harder, but because the body recognizes support.

The Role of Environment

Posture does not exist in isolation. Chairs, screens, counters, beds, and routines all influence how much effort it takes to maintain posture. When the environment demands compensation, the body adapts—often at the cost of comfort.

> A poorly placed screen invites neck strain.

> A chair without support encourages collapse.

> Long periods without movement require bracing.

I remember when I got my piano and spent the first of many hours practicing. The first day, I felt a little discomfort. The second day, that discomfort had morphed into tremendous shoulder pain. When I corrected the height of the bench I was sitting on, though, all the pain I had been in had disappeared by the next day. That proved to me how important posture is in pain.

Pain is often blamed on the body when the environment is the real strain. Supporting alignment sometimes means adjusting the world rather than correcting yourself.

Posture and the Nervous System

Posture is inseparable from the nervous system. A collapsed posture often accompanies fatigue, shutdown, or overwhelm. A rigid posture often reflects vigilance, fear, or hyper-control. Neither is wrong, but both are signals.

When posture is allowed to soften without collapse—upright but not rigid—the nervous system receives a message of safety. Breath deepens. Muscles release. Awareness expands. This is regulation through embodiment.

The Emotional Weight of Alignment

Posture affects more than muscles. Breath changes with alignment. Energy shifts. Emotional state responds.

Try this little experiment: slump heavily and notice how your breathing becomes more difficult. Now sit up straight and pull your shoulders back into alignment with your body, and notice how much easier it is to breathe.

I've noticed that when I sit or stand with gentle alignment, my mood lifts slightly. I feel calmer. More grounded. More capable. The change is subtle, but very real. This has a physiological explanation.

When posture collapses forward, the rib cage compresses, and the diaphragm—the primary muscle of breathing—cannot descend fully. Breath becomes shallow and upper-chest dominant. Shallow breathing signals the nervous system to remain slightly alert. Heart rate variability decreases. Oxygen exchange becomes less efficient. Blood pressure rises. Over time, this pattern can reinforce low energy, anxiety, and even feelings of discouragement.

When the spine is stacked and the rib cage is free to expand, the diaphragm can move more fully. Breath deepens. The vagus nerve—an essential part of the parasympathetic nervous system—receives signals of safety. Heart rhythm stabilizes. Muscles soften. The brain interprets this pattern as reduced threat. Calm increases not because you forced yourself to relax, but because your body was given structural support to do so. This is why deep breathing that has a slower exhale than inhale is so powerful for lowering blood pressure.

Posture does not just reflect emotion. It influences it. Posture reminds me that the body and emotions are not separate systems—they are in constant conversation. Others often respond to posture as well—not because confidence is being performed, but because presence is being embodied.

Pain as Communication, Not Failure

Pain is not always a problem to solve.

Often, it is a message.

Discomfort is the body asking for attention before something escalates. The message may be:

rest

movement

a position change

less intensity

more support

Many of us were taught to override pain—to minimize it, push through it, or treat it as an inconvenience. That pattern erodes trust. When the body learns it will be ignored, it speaks louder.

Learning to pause when pain appears has been one of the most important shifts in my relationship with my body. Instead of immediately asking how to get rid of discomfort, I ask what it might be pointing to.

More often than not, a small response—stretching, standing, shifting posture, resting—prevents pain from becoming chronic. Listening early is an act of prevention.

Chronic Pain and the Cost of Endurance

Chronic pain often begins as unaddressed tension. The body can compensate for a long time, but doing so comes at a cost. When small signals are ignored, muscles overwork. Joints absorb excess load. Breathing becomes restricted. Pain becomes persistent.

Endurance is often praised. But endurance without listening becomes self-betrayal. Pain prevention is not about doing more exercises. It is about responding sooner.

Posture as Presence

Posture becomes powerful when intention is added. Standing or sitting with awareness changes how we show up. It affects how we speak, how we listen, and how we enter a room. Alignment becomes less about appearance and more about embodiment.

When I choose to sit or stand with intention, I feel more present. More self-assured without forcing confidence. My voice steadies. My attention sharpens. Alignment becomes a quiet expression of self-respect. This is not about performing strength. It is about inhabiting your body with care.

Small Shifts, Long-Term Impact

Pain prevention rarely requires dramatic intervention.

It grows out of consistent, small choices:

> noticing tension before it hardens
>
> resetting posture without judgment
>
> responding to discomfort instead of overriding it
>
> allowing alignment to support breath and ease

Over time, these choices accumulate. The body learns it does not need to brace constantly. Muscles release sooner. Pain becomes less frequent. Presence becomes more accessible. Alignment is not about fixing yourself. It is about cooperating with the body you already have.

Carrying Yourself Differently

How we carry our bodies reflects how we relate to ourselves. When posture is treated as self-respect rather than self-correction, something shifts. Movement becomes gentler. Pain becomes more informative. Confidence becomes quieter and more stable.

This week is not about changing everything at once. It is about noticing one tension pattern. Making one small adjustment. Offering your body support instead of endurance. Because how you carry yourself matters—not just for comfort, but for how fully you inhabit your life.

Journal Prompts

Where does my body most often hold tension?

Notice specific areas—jaw, shoulders, hips, lower back, chest.

When does that tension tend to increase?

What is usually happening emotionally or mentally in those moments?

What might my posture be protecting me from?

When I slump, brace, or tighten, what feels vulnerable?

Is my body trying to make me smaller, more alert, less noticeable, more prepared?

What does that tell me about safety?

What changes when I gently realign rather than forcefully correct?

Take a moment to sit or stand with supportive alignment—stacked spine, relaxed shoulders, steady breath.

How does my breathing shift? My mood? My sense of presence?

Where in my life am I enduring instead of adjusting?

Posture often mirrors life patterns.

Is there an area where I am bracing, pushing through, or compensating rather than responding early and kindly?

What would it mean to carry myself with self-respect rather than self-correction?

If alignment were an expression of worth instead of discipline, how would I sit, stand, and move differently this week?

Chapter 9 — Building Strong Bones

Strong bones and healthy joints are not built in moments of effort. They are quietly shaped over time by daily choices that support resilience, mobility, and longevity. We tend to think of skeletal health only when something goes wrong. A knee stiffens. A hip aches. A shoulder complains after years of loyalty. Pain draws attention in a way comfort never does. But bones and joints are always responding—adapting to how we move, how we nourish ourselves, how we rest, and how we respect our limits.

Caring for bones and joints is not about fear of aging or avoiding weakness. It is about preserving freedom. Freedom to move without constant negotiation. Freedom to participate fully in daily life. Freedom to remain independent and embodied for as long as possible. Skeletal health is not about performance—it is about capacity, dignity, and continuity.

The Living Nature of the Skeletal System

Bones are often described as static structures, but they are anything but static. They are living tissue that constantly remodels in response to stress, nutrition, and movement. Joints, too, are dynamic systems—composed of cartilage, connective tissue, fluid, muscle, and nerve feedback—all working together to allow motion.

What this means is simple but profound: the body is always responding.

Bones become stronger when they are gently challenged and adequately nourished. Joints remain healthy when movement is varied, aligned, and supported by rest. Conversely, bones weaken when underused or deprived, and joints deteriorate when overused, misaligned, or ignored. Skeletal health is cumulative. It reflects not what we do occasionally, but what we do consistently.

Nourishment as Ongoing Support, Not Emergency Intervention

When bone health comes up, the conversation often narrows quickly to supplements. Calcium. Vitamin D. Magnesium. Collagen. While these nutrients play important roles, the body does not experience them in isolation.

The skeletal system depends on context. Whole foods provide minerals, vitamins, fats, proteins, and cofactors that work together. Absorption depends on digestion. Utilization depends on hormonal balance. Retention depends on movement and mechanical stimulus. Hydration supports joint lubrication and nutrient transport. No supplement can replace a supportive internal environment.

I've learned that my body responds best to steady nourishment rather than reactive correction. When I prioritize regular meals, hydration, and foods that leave me feeling grounded rather than inflamed, my joints feel more stable, and my body feels less reactive overall. This approach requires patience. It resists the urge to "fix" problems quickly. But bones and joints respond to rhythm, not urgency. Support works best when it is steady and integrated.

Weight Bearing as Dialogue, Not Domination

Bones strengthen in response to load. This is not optional—it is how the skeletal system knows it is needed. But load does not have to mean intensity. It has to mean an appropriate signal.

Weight-bearing movement tells bones to maintain density. It tells joints to maintain integrity. But that signal must be delivered with alignment, variety, and recovery. Too little stimulus weakens bone. Too much, too often, or poorly aligned stimulus damages joints.

Walking has become one of the most reliable ways I support my skeletal health. It provides a consistent, moderate load without overwhelming my joints, particularly when paired with a weighted vest. Gentle strength work adds additional stimulus while respecting my body's limits. When movement feels aligned, my body responds with cooperation rather than resistance.

Enjoyment matters here more than we often admit. Movement that feels punishing rarely lasts, because it isn't sustainable. Movement that feels supportive becomes repeatable, and repetition—not intensity—is what bones respond to over time.

Joint Health Is About How You Move, Not Just How Much You Move

Joint health is shaped less by workouts and more by movement quality throughout the day. How do you sit? How do you stand? How do you carry weight? How do you rise from a chair? Whether you rush or move deliberately. Whether you brace unnecessarily or allow ease. These patterns influence joint wear far more than most people realize.

Posture, footwear, and habitual movement patterns quietly accumulate into either support or strain. Shoes that destabilize alignment increase joint stress. Chairs that encourage collapse strain the hips and spine. Repetitive movements without variation tax connective tissue. Daily habits matter more than occasional effort.

For me, mindful posture, daily walking, and gentle stretching have become protective practices. I've also learned to pace myself—to resist rushing through movements simply because I can. Slowing down reduces impact. Awareness reduces wear.

Joint protection is not about fragility. It is about stewardship.

Recovery Is Part of Strength

One of the most overlooked aspects of skeletal health is rest. Bones and connective tissue do not strengthen during effort—they strengthen during recovery. Rest allows micro-repair. It allows inflammation to resolve. It allows tissue to adapt. Without adequate recovery, even well-intentioned movement becomes erosion.

This is where many people unknowingly undermine their own resilience. They move consistently but never allow their bodies time to repair. Or they oscillate between overuse and complete withdrawal, never finding rhythm.

Rest is not the absence of care. It is one of its most essential forms.

Learning when to pause, when to vary movement, and when to allow the body to recover protects joints far more effectively than pushing through discomfort ever could.

Listening to Early Signals

The body communicates skeletal needs clearly—if we are willing to listen. Stiffness after sitting. Soreness after repetitive movement. A joint that complains at the same time each day. These are not failures. They are early conversations.

I notice joint needs most clearly through stiffness, especially after long periods of stillness or repetitive tasks. When I respond early—standing, walking, stretching, or changing position—the signals often soften quickly. When I ignore them, they escalate.

Pain is rarely the beginning of a problem. It is usually the result of many ignored messages. Listening early prevents long-term damage. It teaches the body that it does not need to shout to be heard, and it prevents problems from escalating.

The Long View Changes Everything

It is easy to care about bones and joints in theory. It is harder to care about them on ordinary days. Long-term vision helps bridge that gap.

When skeletal health is connected to freedom—the ability to walk without fear, to lift without hesitation, to age without unnecessary limitation—choices feel less restrictive and more meaningful.

For me, caring for my bones and joints is not about optimization. It is about preserving the life I want to keep living. Walking with ease. Standing without negotiation. Participating fully in daily life without constant pain management.

That vision shifts motivation. It moves the focus away from short-term results and toward sustainable care.

Aging Without Surrendering Agency

There is a quiet grief that many people carry around with their aging bodies. Fear of decline. Fear of dependence. Fear of losing autonomy. Caring for bones and joints is one way to resist that fear—not through denial, but through preparation.

Strong bones and healthy joints do not guarantee a pain-free life. But they do increase the odds of independence, resilience, and adaptability. They allow us to meet change with capacity instead of collapse.

This is not about staying young.

It is about staying capable.

Freedom Is Built Slowly

Skeletal health is not dramatic. It does not offer instant feedback or quick validation. It grows through nourishment that supports absorption. Movement that stimulates without overwhelming. Habits that reduce wear. Rest that allows repair. Listening that prevents escalation. None of these choices is flashy, but all of them matter.

Strong bones and healthy joints do not demand perfection. They respond to patience, consistency, and respect. They reward those willing to think long-term in a culture obsessed with immediacy.

Caring for your skeletal system is not about fear. It is about freedom. And freedom—to move, to participate, to remain present in your own life—is worth building slowly.

Journal Prompts

What daily habits are either supporting or straining my bones and joints?

Consider how you sit, stand, walk, lift, rest, and nourish yourself.

Which small patterns feel protective?

Which ones feel depleting over time?

When my body feels stiff, sore, or resistant, how do I usually respond?

Do I push through, ignore it, overcorrect, or listen early?

What might change if I treated those signals as a conversation rather than an inconvenience?

What does "freedom of movement" mean to me personally?

Imagine yourself five, ten, or twenty years from now.

What kinds of movement do you hope to preserve?

What daily choices today support that vision?

Where in my life do I rush movement instead of moving with awareness?

How might slowing down—rising from a chair, climbing stairs, lifting an object—change how my joints feel over time?

What would it look like to approach my skeletal health as stewardship instead of optimization?

How does that shift from urgency to long-term care change my motivation?

Chapter 10 — Core Stability & Pelvic Floor Awareness

There are parts of the body we are taught to strengthen, and parts we are taught to ignore…or definitively given the message that they are unmentionable. The pelvic floor often falls into the second category.

For many people, it is either never mentioned at all or spoken about in hushed, clinical, or awkward tones—usually only after something has gone wrong. It is treated as embarrassing, inappropriate, or purely functional, rather than as a vital part of how the body moves, breathes, and feels safe.

That silence comes at a cost.

Core stability, on the other hand, is often misunderstood as tightness, flatness, or control. We are told to "engage," "brace," or "hold it in," without being taught what support actually feels like. The result is often over-tension, disconnection, and fatigue rather than strength.

True stability is not rigidity. It is responsiveness. And the pelvic floor plays a quiet but essential role in that responsiveness—supporting balance, breath, posture, and movement, while also influencing how safe and supported we feel in our bodies.

This chapter invites awareness versus force. Respect over silence. And a different kind of strength—one that works with the body rather than against it.

Breaking the Silence Around the Pelvic Floor

The pelvic floor is rarely discussed openly, especially in wellness spaces that emphasize appearance or performance. When it is discussed, it is often reduced to problems: leaking, weakness, dysfunction, or framed as something to be "fixed."

What's missing is reverence.

The pelvic floor is not a problem area. It is a foundational one. It is a group of muscles and connective tissue that forms the base of the core, supporting organs, coordinating with breath, stabilizing movement, and responding constantly to changes in pressure, posture, and emotion.

Shame has no place here—but it has been placed here anyway.

Many people learned early to disconnect from this part of the body.

> Cultural discomfort.
>
> Religious silence.
>
> Medical dismissal.
>
> Trauma.
>
> Birth.
>
> Surgery.
>
> Chronic stress.
>
> Diet culture.

All of these can shape how aware—or unaware—we are of this region.

Ignoring the pelvic floor does not make it irrelevant. It makes it work harder without support. Rebuilding awareness is not inappropriate. It is responsible.

Rethinking What "Core Strength" Actually Means

When most people hear "core," they think of the abdominal wall. Tight abs. Flat stomachs. Holding everything in. But the core is a system, not a muscle group.

It includes the diaphragm, the deep abdominal muscles, the back muscles, and the pelvic floor. These structures coordinate constantly. Breath affects pressure. Pressure affects stability. Stability affects movement.

Core engagement is dynamic, not constant. You don't walk around holding your breath all day. Your core shouldn't be held rigidly either.

Supportive engagement happens when the body responds to demand—standing up, lifting, reaching, turning—and then releases when the demand passes. Bracing, on the other hand, is continuous tension. It often comes from fear, control, or habit rather than need.

I notice my core engaging most naturally when I move slowly and intentionally—standing from a chair, carrying groceries, reaching overhead. When I focus on breath and alignment rather than tightening, my body feels more stable, not less. Softening does not mean collapsing. It means allowing coordination.

The Pelvic Floor as a Barometer of Stress and Safety

The pelvic floor responds to far more than movement. It responds to posture. To breath. To emotional load. To stress. To vigilance.

Many people hold tension in this area without realizing it. Clenching becomes habitual—especially during stress, concentration, or anxiety. Over time, this constant gripping leads to fatigue, discomfort, or dysfunction. The body is not malfunctioning when this happens. It is adapting.

I notice my pelvic floor asking for attention most clearly after long periods of sitting or during emotionally stressful moments. There's a sense of fatigue or tension—not sharp pain, but subtle strain. When I slow my breath and consciously release instead of gripping, those sensations often ease. This is not about forcing relaxation. It is about restoring choice. Awareness allows early support rather than reactive fixes. It allows the body to reset before strain becomes chronic.

Breath: The Missing Link in Core Support

Breath is the bridge between stability and ease. When breath is shallow or held, pressure in the core increases unevenly. The pelvic floor either overworks or disengages. When breath moves freely, the core system coordinates naturally.

The diaphragm and pelvic floor move together. As one descends, the other responds. This is why forcing core engagement without attention to breath often backfires. The body tightens, but stability decreases. Fatigue increases. Pain appears. Supportive strength allows breath to move.

When I soften my belly slightly and allow breath to deepen, my core feels more supportive, not less. There is a lift without gripping. Stability without strain. This kind of engagement feels different. It feels available.

Exercises That Support Rather Than Strain

More intensity is not always better. Exercises that build true core and pelvic floor support tend to be slower, more controlled, and more intentional. They prioritize awareness, coordination, and quality of movement.

Gentle strength work. Controlled transitions. Intentional stretching. These movements allow the core system to engage as designed—responding to load, adjusting to breath, and releasing when appropriate.

I've learned that when I prioritize quality over quantity, my body responds with ease. When I chase intensity, tension follows.

Supportive exercises don't leave you depleted. They leave you more connected. This approach is especially important for anyone with a history of injury, trauma, chronic stress, or pelvic floor dysfunction. The goal is not to overpower the body, but to restore communication.

Reclaiming Relationship with the Pelvic Area

For many people, the pelvic area carries more than muscle memory. It carries cultural messages. Silence. Shame. Trauma. Neglect. Many of us were taught not to think about this part of the body at all—except in moments of crisis. Others were taught to control it tightly, to hide sensation, to disconnect.

Healing includes reclaiming connection and respect.

Over time, my relationship with my core and pelvic area has shifted. I moved from ignoring or over-tightening to treating it as a supportive center. Learning to listen—to notice tension and release rather than grip—has changed how safe and grounded I feel in my body. This shift didn't happen through force. It happened through awareness.

Supportive Strength Versus Bracing

Bracing feels rigid. Restrictive. Breathless. Supportive strength feels steady, buoyant, and breathable. There is a sense of lift without strain. Balance without rigidity. Movement without fear.

When I brace, my body feels guarded. Fatigue comes quickly. Breath shortens. When I allow support instead of force, I move with more confidence and less exhaustion. This difference matters beyond movement. Supportive strength is a pattern we carry into life. It influences how we handle stress, boundaries, and uncertainty. Bracing often reflects fear. Support reflects trust.

Why This Conversation Matters

Ignoring the pelvic floor does not protect dignity. It undermines health. Silence allows dysfunction to persist. Shame delays care. Misunderstanding leads to over-tightening when release is needed—or disengagement when support is required.

Talking about the pelvic floor is not inappropriate. It is necessary. It is part of treating the body as whole, intelligent, and worthy of care.

Awareness as an Act of Respect

This chapter is not asking you to obsessively monitor or control your body. It is inviting you to notice. To notice when you are gripping unnecessarily. To notice when breath could support movement. To notice when softening would create more stability, not less.

Awareness replaces force. Respect replaces shame.

Core stability and pelvic floor awareness are not about doing more. They are about doing differently—with attention, patience, and trust. When the body feels supported from the inside, movement becomes easier. Pain decreases. Confidence steadies.

Presence deepens. And strength, real strength, becomes something you inhabit, not something you perform.

Journal Prompts

What messages did I learn—spoken or unspoken—about this part of my body?

Were they rooted in silence, embarrassment, control, performance, or neglect?

How have those messages shaped my awareness (or lack of awareness) today?

When I think of "core strength," do I imagine bracing or support?

Where in my life do I tend to grip, hold, or over-control, rather than allowing responsiveness?

What do I notice about my breath throughout the day?

Does it feel shallow, held, rushed, or steady? How might deepening or softening my breath change the way my body feels supported?

During stress or concentration, do I notice subtle tension in my pelvic area or lower abdomen?

What happens when I intentionally soften instead of tighten?

What emotions surface when I practice release?

If supportive strength—not rigidity—were my goal, what would change in how I move, sit, lift, or respond to pressure?

What would it feel like to trust stability instead of forcing it?

Chapter 11 — Functional Fitness for Everyday Tasks

Functional fitness is not about sculpting a body for display. It is about preparing a body for living.

Much of modern fitness culture isolates muscles, counts repetitions, and measures success by appearance. But the body does not live in isolation. It moves as a whole—coordinating balance, strength, breath, and awareness to meet the demands of everyday life.

We lift groceries.

We carry laundry.

We reach overhead.

We stand up from a seated position on the floor.

We navigate uneven ground.

We balance, twist, bend, and recover.

When movement supports these realities, strength becomes meaningful. It builds confidence not because the body looks different, but because it works differently. Functional fitness trains the body for the life you are actually living—not the one imagined in a gym mirror.

This chapter invites a shift from exercise as performance to movement as capability. From training for appearance to training for participation. From proving strength to using it.

When Strength Shows Up Unexpectedly

One of the most encouraging aspects of functional fitness is how quietly it reveals itself. Progress doesn't always announce itself during workouts. It shows up later—unexpectedly—when a task that once felt taxing suddenly feels easier. When balance improves without conscious effort. When coordination feels smoother. When the body moves with less hesitation.

I notice this most clearly in ordinary moments. Carrying groceries no longer feels like a negotiation. Standing up from the floor feels more fluid. Reaching for something no longer brings the same caution or strain. These moments remind me that the work I'm doing is translating into real life, not just exercise sessions.

Functional strength builds trust because it proves itself where it matters…in ease, and ease is a form of evidence.

Training Where You Live

Functional fitness does not require special equipment or perfect conditions. In many ways, the home is the most honest training environment there is. Daily routines offer constant opportunities to build strength, balance, and mobility—if we approach them with intention rather than haste. Standing on one foot while brushing teeth. Engaging the core while lifting a basket. Moving slowly and deliberately when reaching or bending.

These moments are not insignificant. They are the repetitions that shape coordination and confidence. I've found that turning daily movements into practice moments makes strength feel integrated rather than separate. Instead of setting aside fitness as a task, it becomes part of how I move through my day.

Consistency grows when movement fits into real life.

Balance as a Skill, Not a Given

Balance is often taken for granted until it is challenged. Yet balance is not a static trait. It is a skill—one that relies on sensory input, coordination, core support, joint stability, and confidence. It responds to practice, attention, and environment.

Practicing balance does not require elaborate drills. It can look as simple as standing on one foot, shifting weight intentionally, and navigating uneven surfaces mindfully. These simple actions train the nervous system to respond more efficiently.

Balance improves not through fear of falling, but through repeated experiences of stability. When balance strengthens, it affects more than movement. It influences confidence. It reduces hesitation. It allows the body to trust itself again.

Lifting as a Relationship with Gravity

Lifting is one of the most common—and misunderstood—functional tasks. We lift objects every day: bags, boxes, children, furniture, groceries. Yet many people approach lifting with fear, rigidity, or poor mechanics learned through urgency rather than instruction.

Functional fitness reframes lifting as a coordinated movement involving breath, alignment, and support. The goal is not brute force. It is efficiency.

Learning to lift with awareness—using legs, engaging the core dynamically, breathing through effort—reduces strain and builds confidence. It teaches the body that weight is something to work with, not against. When lifting feels safer, life feels less restricted.

Flexibility That Serves Function

Flexibility is often pursued as an aesthetic goal or an extreme one. But functional flexibility is about access—not performance. It is the ability to reach, bend, twist, and recover without hesitation or pain. It allows the body to adapt to unexpected demands without injury.

Functional flexibility grows through gentle range-of-motion work, varied movement, and listening to limits rather than forcing past them. It supports joints by allowing movement to distribute load rather than concentrate it. When flexibility serves function, it enhances confidence rather than demanding comparison.

Motivation Rooted in Real Life

Sustainable motivation rarely comes from abstract goals. It comes from meaning.

For me, the motivation behind functional fitness is simple and profound: I want to move confidently and independently—now and in the future. I want my body to support my life rather than limit it. That vision keeps me engaged even when motivation dips.

Real-life goals are often relational. Being present. Being capable. Being able to participate fully. When movement serves these goals, it becomes supportive rather than obligatory. Purpose sustains effort better than pressure ever could.

When Difficulty Becomes Information

Functional fitness does not eliminate challenge. It clarifies it.

Certain tasks still challenge me—reaching overhead, getting up from the floor, maintaining stability during transitions. But instead of discouragement, these moments now offer guidance.

Difficulty is information. It highlights where mobility, strength, or coordination could be supported further. It points toward areas that need patience rather than judgment. Approaching challenges with curiosity transforms frustration into learning. It keeps the relationship with the body intact even when progress is slow.

Capability and Identity

As the body becomes more capable, something shifts internally. Confidence grows—not the loud kind, but the grounded kind. A sense of agency emerges. The body feels less like something to manage and more like something to rely on.

Becoming more capable has changed how I see myself. I feel steadier. More secure. More appreciative of what my body offers me daily. This confidence is not about appearance. It is about trust.

Capability reshapes identity. It changes how we move through the world—not with bravado, but with presence.

Celebrating Function Over Form

Functional fitness invites a different kind of celebration. Not before-and-after photos. Not numbers on a chart. But moments of ease. Moments of confidence. Moments when the body supports life quietly and effectively.

Celebrating function reinforces what truly matters. It aligns effort with values. It honors progress that cannot always be measured but can always be felt. When function is celebrated, the body is no longer pressured to perform for approval. It is valued for participation.

Resilience Built Through Relevance

Functional fitness builds resilience because it trains what is actually needed. It prepares the body for unpredictability. For uneven surfaces. For fatigue. For real-world demands that don't arrive neatly packaged.

Resilience is not about being unbreakable. It is about being adaptable. Training the body to respond to real life builds confidence that extends beyond movement. It reinforces the belief that you can meet what comes—not perfectly, but competently.

Living in a Capable Body

Functional fitness is not flashy.

> It is practical.

> It is dignified.

> It is deeply empowering.

It restores trust not by promising transformation, but by delivering support where it matters most. It allows strength to be lived, not displayed.

When the body can support daily life with less effort and more confidence, health stops being a project and becomes a partnership. And that partnership—between intention and ability, between care and capacity—is what allows the body to truly support the life you are living.

Journal Prompt:

What everyday task feels easier for me now than it did in the past?

How does that change affect my confidence or sense of independence?

Where in my daily life could I turn ordinary movement into intentional practice?

(Standing, lifting, balancing, reaching, carrying.)

What would it look like to move with awareness instead of rushing?

When I encounter difficulty in a physical task, how do I interpret it?

Do I see it as a failure, a limitation, or information?

What might change if I approached it with curiosity instead of judgment?

What does "capability" mean to me at the stage of life I am currently in?

How is that different from appearance-based goals I may have held in the past?

If I imagine my future self 10–20 years from now, what kind of physical freedom do I hope to preserve?

What small, consistent practices today support that vision?

Chapter 12 — Community & Reflection: Seeing Yourself Through Healthy Connections

There comes a point in any healing journey where the most radical act is not effort, but pause. Not stopping because you are tired or overwhelmed, but stopping because something has shifted—and it deserves to be noticed.

This chapter is that pause.

Along this journey, strength has been redefined. Trust has been rebuilt. Movement has shifted from obligation to relationship. The body has gone from something to manage to something to partner with. And now, rather than rushing ahead to the next goal, this chapter invites you to turn toward what is already here.

> To notice.

> To honor.

> To celebrate.

Because bodies do not heal loudly. They heal quietly, in small returns of ease, confidence, and presence that are easy to miss if we are always looking ahead.

True beauty lives in those quiet victories.

The Abilities We Once Took for Granted

There are things the body does so faithfully that we rarely notice them—until they become difficult or disappear.

Standing up without hesitation.

Walking without pain.

Carrying a bag.

Reaching overhead.

Moving through a day without constant negotiation.

These abilities often fade gradually and return just as quietly.

I once took it for granted that I could move through my day with ease. When pain entered the picture, that ease became something I longed for rather than assumed. Now, moments of comfort feel like gifts. Each day with less pain is a reminder of how resilient and responsive the body can be when it is supported rather than fought.

Recovery rarely announces itself. It shows up in ordinary moments. Recovery may look like a smoother transition, a steadier step, or a calmer nervous system. Awareness transforms these moments from background noise into gratitude.

Loss sharpens appreciation.

Recovery deepens it.

Strength Learned Through Living

Cultural definitions of strength are loud and narrow. They reward pushing, proving, and enduring. They often confuse intensity with capability and mistake appearance with power. But lived experience tells a different story.

Real strength is learned over time, through injury, fatigue, adaptation, and humility. It reveals itself not in how much we can override, but in how well we can respond.

My definition of strength has changed dramatically. It used to mean pushing through discomfort and ignoring signals. Now, strength feels like adaptability—knowing when to move forward and when to rest without guilt. It feels like discernment. Like staying connected instead of being checked out. This kind of strength does not perform well on social media. It does not seek applause. But it does sustain life.

Strength evolves with seasons. What was once necessary may later be harmful. What once felt weak may later reveal itself as wisdom. Allowing that to evolve is in itself a mark of maturity.

Feeling at Home in the Body

Many people move through life feeling like guests, or worse, strangers in their own bodies—monitoring, evaluating, correcting, but never settling. Feeling "at home" in the body is not about loving every aspect of it. It is about safety. Acceptance. Presence. It is about no longer bracing for judgment—from yourself or from others.

I feel most at home in my body during unguarded moments. Gentle movement outdoors. Rest without urgency. Breathing without effort. In those moments, there is no internal commentary, no measuring, no comparison. Just being.

Belonging begins internally. When the body feels safe enough to be inhabited, the need to perform softens. Comfort becomes possible—not because everything is perfect, but because the relationship is intact.

Feeling "at home" is not a destination. It is a way of relating.

Participation Over Performance

The body is not meant to be admired in isolation. It is meant to enable participation. It allows us to show up for work, for loved ones, for responsibilities, and the joys that give life meaning. It carries us into rooms, conversations, relationships, and moments that matter.

Performance asks how we look while doing something, but participation asks whether we can be there at all.

My motivation to care for my body is rooted in this truth. I want to participate fully. To engage without constant limitation. To say yes to what matters without fear of what it will cost my body later.

Gratitude deepens when we recognize how much the body enables. Even on hard days. Even with limitations. Participation is not about doing everything—it is about being present where you are. That presence is a form of beauty.

Beauty Beyond Comparison

Comparison thrives on narrow definitions. It requires standards, hierarchies, and constant evaluation. Beauty defined by appearance alone is fragile—it rises and falls with trends, age, and circumstance.

Beauty rooted in function is different. It is enduring. It is expansive. It allows for variation, seasonality, and individuality. When beauty is defined by capability, presence, and vitality, it becomes something we inhabit rather than chase.

Honoring what the body can do reframes self-worth. Appreciation replaces assessment. Comparison loses its grip because the metric has changed.

When I view my body through the lens of ability rather than appearance, beauty feels less restrictive. It becomes about aliveness. Responsiveness. Participation. Experience.

This kind of beauty cannot be standardized. And that is its strength.

The Quiet Victories

Not all victories are dramatic. Some are almost invisible: fewer aches, steadier energy, calmer responses, quicker recovery. These changes do not demand recognition, but they do deserve it.

Celebration does not require fanfare. It requires noticing. Pausing to acknowledge what is working builds trust. It reinforces the relationship you have been rebuilding with your body. It signals that progress is not only allowed, but valued—even when it is subtle. Quiet victories accumulate. They form the foundation of sustainable health.

Redefining What It Means to Be Strong and Beautiful

Strength is no longer about domination.

Beauty is no longer about conformity.

Together, they form something richer: embodiment.

An embodied body is not perfect. It is present. It participates. It adapts. It carries history and possibility at the same time. Honoring your body's abilities does not mean denying struggle. It means refusing to define yourself solely by limitation. It means allowing appreciation to coexist with effort.

This redefinition is not theoretical. It is lived—in how you move, how you rest, how you speak to yourself, and how you allow your body to take up space.

Celebration as Integration

Celebration is not the end of the journey. It is how the journey integrates. By celebrating what your body can do, you anchor change in gratitude rather than pressure. You reinforce that health is not about arriving somewhere else, but about living more fully where you are.

This chapter is an invitation to mark what has shifted. To recognize who you have become. To honor the body that has carried you here—still learning, still adapting, still showing up. The work does not disappear after this point. But it becomes lighter. Less adversarial. More relational. And that, perhaps, is the most beautiful outcome of all.

Carrying This Forward

As you move beyond this chapter, the invitation is simple:

> Notice what works.

> Honor what has returned.

> Celebrate what is possible.

> Let strength remain flexible.

Let beauty remain broad.

Let your body remain a place you can live—not just manage.

Because the most enduring transformation is not how you look when you move. It is how fully you can participate in your life.

Journal Prompt:

What is something my body can do today that I once struggled with or took for granted?

How does it feel to acknowledge that ability now?

Where have I noticed quiet victories in this journey?

(Examples: steadier energy, less pain, calmer reactions, greater ease in daily tasks.)

What would change if I allowed myself to celebrate these fully?

How has my definition of strength evolved over the past 12 weeks?

What does strength mean to me now — in my body and in my life?

When do I feel most "at home" in my body?

What conditions, practices, or environments help me feel present rather than self-conscious?

If I shift my focus from performance to participation, what becomes possible for me?

Where do I want my body to support fuller participation in my life moving forward?

About R.I.S.E.

R.I.S.E. was created as a place of encouragement, clarity, and support for those choosing a whole food plant-based lifestyle and seeking to live in whole-being wellness. It is a framework for living that honors the Creator's original design for the body, mind, and spirit.

R.I.S.E. means:

Rooted in Truth – grounded in unshakable principles rather than passing trends.

Intentional in Habits – choosing daily practices that nourish and strengthen both body and soul.

Strong in Spirit – cultivating inner resilience, emotional stability, and faith for life's challenges.

Energized for Life – experiencing vibrancy, joy, and well-being through alignment, simplicity, and purpose.

Through R.I.S.E., you'll discover tools, teachings, and community support that help you walk toward wholeness with confidence. It's not only about food—it's about restoring balance, reclaiming identity, living with intention, and stepping into the fullness of life you were created for.

Every resource connected to R.I.S.E., including this book and companion journal, is designed to equip, uplift, and inspire you as you grow in wellness and walk out your calling with clarity and courage.

Feel free to reach out anytime to learn more about R.I.S.E. using the QR code below.

About the Author

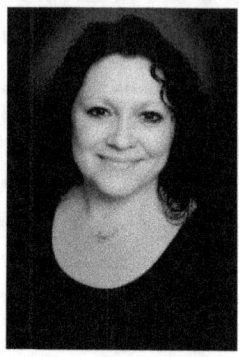

Angel Tate Keaton is the founder of Healthy in Heart Media and the creator of the RISE™ Rooted, Intentional, Strong, Energized, a Whole-Being Wellness Framework. As a trauma survivor, teacher, author, and guide, Angel writes from the intersections of faith, identity, emotional healing, and whole-being restoration. Her work invites others to remember who they are beneath the labels, lies, and lifetimes of survival—and to step into the truth of who they were created to become.

After decades of healing work, Angel discovered that transformation doesn't begin with performance, perfection, or self-improvement—it starts with identity. This book and companion journal reflect her heart: to help others move from wounded stories to whole stories, from exhaustion to alignment, and from fractured self-image to beloved self-understanding. Through simple prompts, gentle questions, and the RISE rhythm of weekly reflection, she invites readers into a deeper clarity with a grounded confidence.

Angel believes that every person carries divine worth and that healing unfolds not by running faster but by returning to truth. Her mission is to create resources that help individuals rebuild their identity, release shame, reclaim resilience, and rise with purpose—spiritually, emotionally, and physically. Through books, journals, guides, community circles, and teaching, she is dedicated to supporting others in living lives rooted in truth, intentional in purpose, strong in identity, and energized in spirit.

Angel lives in Virginia with her husband, Todd, and their daughter, where they continue to write, teach, and walk out whole-being living with a shared passion for helping others rediscover the path back to themselves—and back to the One who made them.

Mission of Healthy in Heart

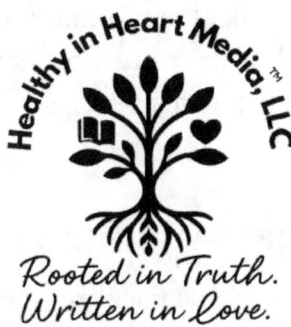

Healthy in Heart Media, LLC exists to help people return to wholeness—body, mind, and spirit—through Hebraic truth, Eden-aligned living, and compassionate, practical tools.

We:

- Publish books, journals, devotionals, and children's resources that make spiritual formation simple and doable.
- Guide households into oil-free, whole-food, plant-based eating through meal plans, prep systems, and gentle re-entry guides.
- Cultivate Sabbath and seasonal practices that restore pace, presence, and peace.

Mission in one line:

To restore shalom in real lives through truth, tools, and tables—so homes and communities become a little piece of Eden.

Join the Healthy in Heart Community

Wholeness is not a journey we walk alone. If this book has strengthened your spirit, I invite you to stay connected with a growing community that is learning and returning to whole-being wellness together.

Visit the Healthy in Heart Website

Find more books, journals, recipes, botanical resources, and tools for whole-being wellness.

Website: HealthyInHeart.com

Follow Along on Social Media

Receive weekly encouragement, recipe ideas, spiritual reflections, and behind-the-scenes updates on upcoming projects.

YouTube | Instagram| Facebook

@healthyinheart

Pinterest

@healthyinheart1

Join the Sabbath Table Gathering

A weekly space of peace, Scripture, reflection, shared learning, and social connection.

We gather to slow down, honor the rhythm God built into creation, and get to know one another. We talk about whatever subject comes up.

Everyone is welcome — whether you're exploring Sabbath for the first time or restoring it in your home. To request an invite:

https://healthyinheart.com/contact-me-about-our-sabbath-table-gathering

The RISE™ Momentum Circle

If you desire deeper transformation, the RISE Circle offers guided group discussion rooted in whole-being wellness:

Rooted • Intentional • Strong • Energized

Together we grow in identity, emotional strength, nourishing rhythms, and whole-being wellness.

We meet on Zoom on Thursdays from 5:00 PM to 6:30 PM. To request an invite:

https://healthyinheart.com/contact-me-about-r-i-s-e

Stay Connected

Subscribe to the Healthy in Heart newsletter email list for free resources, new recipes, devotional content, early book releases, and special community invitations.

https://healthyinheart.com/subscribe

You don't have to walk toward wholeness alone.

Join us — and step into a community shaped by truth, simplicity, joy, and shalom.

Explore More

Your journey doesn't have to end here. If these pages have spoken to you, I'd love to walk further with you. My online store is filled with resources created to nourish your identity, strengthen your spirit, and support whole-being wellness—books that deepen your walk, journals that guide your reflection, themed shirts and home goods that encourage you daily, and handmade items crafted with prayer and purpose.

Every product is designed to remind you of who you are and Who walks with you. Come see what's waiting for you at **HealthyInHeart.com**

Shop Healthy in Heart Store

Each week, I release new blog articles and plant-based recipes designed to support your health, healing, identity, and whole-being wellness. From emotional and spiritual encouragement to practical nourishment for your body, these writings are meant to walk with you—one small step at a time.

You'll find teachings on R.I.S.E. principles, identity and worth, emotional healing, Hebraic roots, and simple homemade recipes that help you thrive.

Join me at HealthyInHeart.com for weekly encouragement, truth, and nourishment for both body and soul. Subscribe to my newsletter by following this QR code where you can keep up-to-date on my most recent posts, new books, and monthly updates.

Sign up for the Newsletter!

The Healthy in Heart Library

The Daniel Fast 21-Day Meal Plan: Simple Plant-Based Nourishment for Mind, Body, & Spirit Eat Well. Pray Deep. Stand Strong.

Creation Needs the Sabbath: Time That Heals Was Never Just For Jews

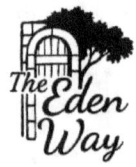

Books in the Series

Book 1- *The Eden Way*™*: Reclaiming Body, Mind, and Spirit Through the Creator's Original Design*

Book 2 -*The Eden Way*™ *Journal: 49-Days to Reset Body, Mind, and Spirit* (Companion to Book 1)

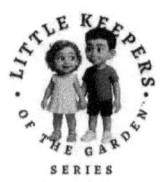

Books in the Series

The Little Keepers of the Garden™*: Seeds of Truth Collection*

Seeds of Truth Activity Book: The Little Keepers of the Garden™ *Series*

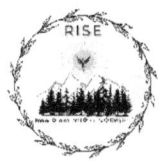

Books in the Series

RISE™ Wellness Journal—Rooted, Intentional, Strong, Energized: Embrace One Year of Habits, Healing, and Hope

RISE™ The Beginning of Balance—How Rooted, Intentional, Strong, and Energized Living Transforms the Whole Self: A Framework for Whole-Being Wellness

The Beginning of Balance Chronicles: The Lived Record of Learning to Inhabit RISE™

The RISE™ Circle of Wholeness Collection

Identity & Worth Volume 1

RISE™ Identity & Worth Living a Rooted, Intentional, Strong, and Energized Life—Volume 1

RISE™ Identity & Worth Journal: A 12-Week Journey to a Rooted, Intentional, Strong, and Energized Life—Volume 1 (Companion to Identity & Worth, Volume 1)

Body Trust, Movement, & Mindful Strength Volume 2

RISE™ Body Trust, Movement, & Mindful Strength: Living a Rooted, Intentional, Strong, and Energized Life — through Embodied Strength and Trust Volume 2

RISE™ Body Trust, Movement, & Mindful Strength Journal: A 12-Week Journey Toward Embodied Strength and Trust Volume 2

Explore all titles and resources at HealthyInHeart.com

If This Book Spoke to You...

A Note from the Author

If this journey has nourished your body, quieted old patterns, renewed your mind, or gently drawn you closer to God through simplicity and intention, thank you for walking it with me.

Books like this find their way into the right hands not just through algorithms, but through shared stories. When readers take a moment to reflect publicly—whether in a few sentences or a single honest thought—it becomes a signpost for someone else seeking the same clarity, healing, or rest.

Your words matter more than you know.

They help others recognize themselves in this path.

They remind someone that restoration is possible.

If you feel led, I would be deeply grateful if you shared a brief review wherever you normally discover books—Amazon, Goodreads, or HealthyInHeart.com.

Thank you for choosing nourishment over noise, truth over striving, and faithfulness over perfection.

And thank you for helping this message reach those who are longing to return to what is whole.

With gratitude,

Angel Tate Keaton